BRITISH MEDICAL BULLETIN
VOLUME 67   2003

Preg

Reducing maternal death and disability

Scientific Editor

Charles Rodeck

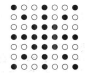

OXFORD
UNIVERSITY PRESS

PUBLISHED FOR THE BRITISH COUNCIL BY
OXFORD UNIVERSITY PRESS

OXFORD UNIVERSITY PRESS
Great Clarendon Street, Oxford OX2 6DP, UK

British Library Cataloguing in Publication Data
A catalogue record for this book is available from the British Library
ISBN 0-19-8526997-2
ISSN 0007–1420

Subscription information *British Medical Bulletin* is published quarterly on behalf of The British Council. Subscription rates for 2003 are £185/$315 for four volumes, each of one issue. Prices include distribution; the British Medical Bulletin is distributed by surface mail within Europe, by air freight and second class post within the USA*, and by various methods of air-speeded delivery to all other countries. Subscription orders, single issue orders and enquiries regarding volumes from 2001 onwards should be sent to:

Oxford University Press, Great Clarendon Street, Oxford OX2 6DP, UK (Tel +44 (0)1865 353907; Fax +44(0)1865 353485; E-mail: jnl.orders@oup.co.uk

*Periodicals postage paid at Rahway, NJ. US Postmaster: Send address changes to *British Medical Bulletin*, c/o Mercury Airfreight International Ltd, 365 Blair Road, Avenel, NJ 07001, USA.

Back numbers of titles published 1996–2000 are available from The Royal Society of Medicine Press Limited, 1 Wimpole St, London W1G 0AE, UK. (Tel. +44 (0)20 7290 2921; Fax +44 (0)20 7290 2929); www.rsm.ac.uk/pub/bmb/htm).

Pre-1996 back numbers: Contact Jill Kettley, Subscriptions Manager, Harcourt Brace, Foots Cray, Sidcup, Kent DA14 5HP (Tel +44 (0)20 8308 5700; Fax +44 (0)20 8309 0807).

This journal is indexed, abstracted and/or published online in the following media: Adonis, Biosis, BRS Colleague (full text), Chemical Abstracts, Colleague (Online), Current Contents/Clinical Medicine, Current Contents/Life Sciences, Elsevier BIOBASE/Current Awareness in Biological Sciences, EMBASE/Excerpta Medica, Index Medicus/Medline, Medical Documentation Service, Reference Update, Research Alert, Science Citation Index, Scisearch, SIIC-Database Argentina, UMI (Microfilms)

Printed in Great Britain by Bell & Bain Ltd, Glasgow, Scotland.

Pregnancy

Reducing maternal death and disability

Scientific Editor: Charles Rodeck

http://www.bmb.oupjournals.org

Acknowledgements

The planning committee for this issue of the British Medical Bulletin was chaired by Charles Rodeck and also included Professor James Drife, Professor Marion Hall, Professor James Neilson and Dr Gwynneth Lewis

The British Council and Oxford University Press are most grateful to the Scientific Editors for their expert assistance in the completion of this volume. Special thanks are also extended to Nancy Durrell McKenna, Executive Director of Safe-Hands Charitable Trust for providing the cover image.

Material Disclaimer

Drug Disclaimer

Global burden of maternal death and disability

Carla AbouZahr

World Health Organization, Geneva, Switzerland

Sound information is the prerequisite for health action: without data on the dimensions, impact and significance of a health problem it is neither possible to create an advocacy case nor to establish strong programmes for addressing it. The absence of good information on the extent of the burden of maternal ill-health resulted in its relative neglect by the international health community for many years. Maternal deaths are too often solitary and hidden events that go uncounted. The difficulty arises not because of lack of clarity regarding the definition of a maternal death, but because of the weakness of health information systems and consequent absence of the systematic identification and recording of maternal deaths. In recent years, innovative approaches to measuring maternal mortality have been developed, resulting in a stronger information base. WHO, UNICEF and UNFPA estimates for the year 2000 indicate that most of the total 529,000 maternal deaths globally occur in just 13 countries. By contrast, information on the global burden of non-fatal health outcomes associated with pregnancy and childbearing remains patchy and incomplete. Nonetheless, initial estimates based on systematic reviews of available information and confined to the five major direct pregnancy-related complications indicate a problem of considerable magnitude.

Introduction

Correspondence to:
Carla AbouZahr,
Coordinator, Advocacy,
Communications and
Evaluation, Office of the
Executive Director,
Family and Community
Health, World Health
Organization,
20 Avenue Appia, CH-1211
Geneva 27, Switzerland.
E-mail: abouzahrc@
who.int

One of the reasons why maternal mortality was a neglected problem for so long was inadequate information. Countries with the highest levels of mortality seldom have good coverage or reporting of vital events such as births and deaths. And even countries with relatively complete vital registration (generally defined as covering some 90% of the population) may have less than adequate attribution of causes of death. This is important because in order to decide whether the death of a women is a maternal death or not it is essential to know both the timing of the death in relation to the pregnancy status of the woman and the cause of death. Herein lies one of the biggest challenges when it comes to measuring the dimensions of the burden of maternal mortality and morbidity.

Measurement challenges

The Tenth Revision of the International Classification of Diseases (ICD-10) defines a maternal death as the death of a woman while pregnant or within 42 days of termination of pregnancy, irrespective of the duration and site of the pregnancy, from any cause related to or aggravated by the pregnancy or its management but not from accidental or incidental causes[1]. There are two problems with this definition, one related to time of death, the second to cause of death. With regard to the first, historically, maternal mortality was defined as deaths occurring within 6 weeks of termination of pregnancy. Modern life-sustaining procedures and technologies can, however, prolong dying and delay death. Even before the era of modern medicine it is likely that some maternal deaths took place beyond the 6 week interval, but the proportion was probably very small. Medical procedures may increase that proportion, but it is likely to remain fairly small though by no means negligible. For example, the Centers for Disease Control reports that 29% of maternal deaths in Georgia, USA, over the period 1974–75 occurred after 42 days of pregnancy termination and 6% occurred after 90 days post-partum[2].

The second problem with the definition of maternal death lies in the classification of cause of death. The drawback is that maternal deaths can escape being so classified because the precise cause of death cannot be given even though the fact of the woman having been pregnant is known. Such under-registration is frequent in both developing and developed countries. Even in countries where all or most deaths are medically certified, maternity-related mortality can still be grossly underestimated. Record linking and other studies have shown misreporting of between 25% and 70% of maternal deaths[3,4].

According to ICD-9 and ICD-10, maternal deaths should be divided into two groups: *direct obstetric deaths* resulting from obstetric complications of the pregnant state (pregnancy, labour and the puerperium); and *indirect obstetric deaths* resulting from previous existing disease or disease that developed during pregnancy and which was aggravated by the physiologic effects of pregnancy. Indirect maternal deaths are particularly prone to being reported as non-maternal and there are significant differences between countries in the classification of indirect deaths to the maternal category. Of the 60 countries reporting vital registration figures for causes of maternal deaths over the period 1992–1993, over half (33 countries) reported no indirect deaths at all. Yet the 1997–99 Confidential Enquiry in the UK found that indirect deaths now account for more maternal deaths than deaths due to direct causes[5].

Deaths from 'accidental or incidental' causes have historically been excluded from maternal mortality. However, in practice, the distinction between incidental and indirect causes of death is difficult to make. Some deaths from external causes may be attributable to the pregnancy itself. It is likely that many homicides and suicides of pregnant or recently pregnant women are attributable in some way to the pregnancy[6,7]. In practice, different countries use different definitions and this renders it difficult to make comparisons between countries about the dimensions and patterns of maternal mortality.

Global estimates of maternal mortality

The difficulty of measuring maternal mortality has long been an impediment to progress in alerting health planners and others to the magnitude and causes of the problem and hence to effective interventions on an appropriate scale. In order to strengthen the information base, WHO, UNICEF and UNFPA have developed an approach to estimating maternal mortality that seeks both to generate estimates for countries with no data and to correct available data for underreporting and misclassification. A dual strategy is used which involves adjusting available country data and developing a simple model to generate estimates for countries without reliable information. Inevitably, given the uncertainty of the available data, the estimates are subject to wide margins of uncertainty and cannot be used to monitor short-term trends. In addition, cross-country comparisons should be treated with considerable circumspection because different strategies are used to derive the estimates for different countries, rendering comparisons fraught with difficulty. Nonetheless, the approach, with some variations, was used to develop estimates for maternal mortality in 1990, 1995 and 2000[8].

The estimated number of maternal deaths in 2000 for the world was 529,000 (Table 1). These deaths were almost equally divided between Africa (251,000) and Asia (253,000), with about 4% (22,000) occurring in Latin America and the Caribbean, and less than 1% (2500) in the more developed regions of the world. In terms of the maternal mortality ratio (MMR), the world figure is estimated to be 400 per 100,000 live births. By region, the MMR was highest in Africa (830), followed by Asia (330), Oceania (240), Latin America and the Caribbean (190), and the developed countries (20).

The country with the highest estimated number of maternal deaths is India (136,000), followed by Nigeria (37,000), Pakistan (26,000), Democratic Republic of Congo and Ethiopia (24,000 each), the United Republic of Tanzania (21,000), Afghanistan (20,000), Bangladesh (16,000), Angola, China and Kenya (11,000 each), Indonesia and Uganda (10,000 each). These 13 countries account for 67% of all maternal deaths.

Table 1 2000 Maternal mortality estimates by United Nations MDG regions

Region	Maternal mortality ratio (maternal deaths per 100,000 live births)	Number of maternal deaths	Lifetime risk of maternal death, 1 in:
World total	400	529,000	74
Developed regions[a]	20	2500	2800
Europe	24	1700	2400
Developing regions	440	527,000	61
Africa	830	251,000	20
Northern Africa	130	4600	210
Sub-Saharan Africa	920	247,000	16
Asia	330	253,000	94
Eastern Asia	55	11,000	840
South-Central Asia	520	207,000	46
South-Eastern Asia	210	25,000	140
Western Asia	190	9800	120
Latin America & the Caribbean	190	22,000	160
Oceania	240	530	83

[a]Includes Canada, USA, Japan, Australia and New Zealand which are excluded from the regional totals.

However, the number of maternal deaths is the product of the total number of births and obstetric risk per birth, described by the MMR. On a risk per birth basis, the list looks rather different. With the sole exception of Afghanistan, the countries with the highest MMRs are in Africa. The highest MMRs of 1000 or greater are, in rank order, Sierra Leone, Afghanistan, Malawi, Angola, Niger, the United Republic of Tanzania, Rwanda, Mali, Somalia, Zimbabwe, Chad, Central African Republic, Guinea Bissau, Kenya, Mozambique, Burkina Faso, Burundi and Mauritania.

Causes of maternal deaths and disabilities

In calculating the overall burden of ill-health associated with pregnancy and childbirth, it is necessary to estimate the incidence of obstetric complications, their case fatality rates in different settings, and the incidence and severity of non-fatal health outcomes. A comprehensive analysis of the burden of obstetric mortality and morbidity would need to address both direct and indirect causes of deaths and disabilities, and at least some of the incidental causes. Direct conditions would include temporary, mild or severe conditions which occur during pregnancy and within 42 days of delivery (such as haemorrhage, eclampsia or sepsis) or permanent/chronic conditions that persist beyond the puerperium (such as obstetric fistula, urinary or faecal incontinence, scarred uterus, pelvic inflammatory disease, palsy). Indirect conditions would include, for example, anaemia, malaria, hepatitis, tuberculosis and cardiovascular disease. Psychological obstetric morbidity would include puerperal psychoses, post-partum depression (baby blues), suicide, and strong fear of pregnancy and childbirth resulting from, for example, obstetric complications, interventions or cultural practices.

In practice, given the paucity of the data, WHO has developed estimates of mortality and morbidity related to just five direct obstetric conditions: post-partum haemorrhage, puerperal sepsis, pre-eclampsia and eclampsia, obstructed labour and abortion. Non-fatal health outcomes of other direct obstetric complications, such as ectopic and molar pregnancies, anaesthetic complications, cerebrovascular accidents, embolisms, are not included here. Nor are the non-fatal health outcomes of indirect causes of maternal deaths.

A general problem encountered in attempting to estimate incidence of pregnancy-related complications is that the different sources of data are neither representative nor comparable. Hospital statistics indicate the incidence of the condition among women delivering in hospitals, and are therefore reliable only for developed countries, where most deliveries take place in hospitals. On the other hand, self-reported maternal morbidity tends to overestimate incidence and the results very much depend on the sensitivity and specificity of the data collection instruments. Several attempts have been made to validate the results of self-reported maternal morbidity, and some of them compared the results from interviewing women shortly after hospital delivery with hospital case notes. Comparisons are difficult, as studies may have used different definitions and study design, and their results may not be generalized to the population which does not deliver in hospital. Thus, self-reported maternal morbidity cannot provide exact estimates of prevalence and incidence[9].

Given these constraints, estimates of the overall burden of maternal ill-health associated with pregnancy and childbearing are necessarily incomplete. Nonetheless, they provide an idea of the orders of magnitude of the problem. These initial estimates have been developed for WHO's calculations of the global burden of disease and are based upon both literature review and expert consensus. They are currently under review and final results along with details of the methodologies and data sources will be published in the World Health Report.

Maternal haemorrhage

Maternal haemorrhage consists of bleeding from the genital tract during pregnancy (antepartum), during or after the delivery of the infant (intra- and post-partum). Although in developed countries antepartum haemorrhage is no longer a major cause of maternal mortality, it is still an important cause of maternal and perinatal morbidity[10]. In contrast, post-partum haemorrhage continues to be a major cause of maternal death both in

Table 2 Estimated incidence of major obstetric complications and main maternal sequelae (2000)

Complication	Incidence (% of live births)	Cases	Case fatality rate (%)	Maternal deaths 2000	Main sequelae
Severe post-partum haemorrhage	10.5	13,795,000	1.0	132,000	Severe anaemia
Sepsis	4.4	5,768,000	1.3	79,000	Infertility
Pre-eclampsia/ eclampsia	3.2	4,152,000	1.7	63,000	Eclampsia
Obstructed labour	4.6	6,038,000	0.7	42,000	Urinary incontinence, fistula
Abortion	14.8	19,340,000	0.3	69,000	Infertility

the developing as well as in the developed world and we therefore focus on post-partum haemorrhage in these estimates. Although the formal definition of post-partum haemorrhage is blood loss of 500 ml or more within 24 h after delivery and/or within 42 weeks following delivery, we considered only blood loss of 1000 ml or more, because it has greater clinical significance. We considered only one major sequela of severe post-partum haemorrhage, namely anaemia.

On the basis of data convened from a review of published literature, combined with expert consensus, we estimate an incidence of severe post-partum haemorrhage globally of around 10.5% of live births. Clearly, incidence is lower in developed country settings where most women deliver in a hospital and where active management of the third stage of labour is the norm, compared to developing areas where large proportions of women deliver at home. Based on the global average, we estimate that each year nearly 14 million women suffer severe blood loss during childbirth or the post-partum period. We estimate that around 140,000 women die as a result, a case fatality rate of 1%. A further 12% survive but with severe anaemia, meaning that each year, some 1.6 million women of reproductive age suffer from long-lasting and debilitating consequences of anaemia due to pregnancy-related complications (Table 2).

Sepsis

Historically, puerperal sepsis was a common pregnancy-related condition, which could eventually lead to obstetric shock or even death. During the 19th century, it took on epidemic proportions, particularly in lying-in hospitals, where ignorance of asepsis prevailed. The efforts of Wendell Holmes and Semmelweis to improve asepsis during childbirth resulted in a striking decrease in mortality due to puerperal sepsis between 1846 and 1847[11]. With the introduction of antibiotics, puerperal fever declined further in developed countries. Puerperal sepsis is nonetheless still prevalent in developing countries and continues to present a significant risk of obstetric morbidity and mortality. Moreover, nosocomial infections, particularly related to operative deliveries, and antibiotic resistance, are increasingly common in both developed and developing regions[12].

Puerperal infection is a general term used to describe any infection of the genital tract after delivery. Because most pyrexia in the puerperium is caused by pelvic infections, the incidence of fever after childbirth may be a reliable index of their incidence though fever may also be associated with other infections related to childbirth such as mastitis. In the absence of antibiotic treatment or in more severe cases, puerperal infection may be complicated by pelvic chronic pain, pelvic inflammatory disease, bilateral tubal occlusion and infertility.

Estimating the incidence of sepsis around the world is fraught with difficulty because the aetiology and epidemiology of sepsis vary enormously as a result of local conditions, in particular with regard to hygiene during delivery but also as a function of rates of reproductive tract infections, including sexually transmitted infections. Rates of puerperal sepsis are generally higher in settings with high HIV prevalence. Based on a literature review of hospital and community studies, we estimated the incidence of sepsis globally to be 4.4% of live births, giving a total number of puerperal sepsis cases of nearly 6 million and almost 77,000 maternal deaths. The most significant long-term complication is infertility resulting from tubal occlusion, estimated to affect some 450,000 women each year.

Pre-eclampsia and eclampsia

Hypertensive disorders of pregnancy (HDP) represent a group of conditions associated with high blood pressure during pregnancy, proteinuria and in some cases convulsions. The most serious consequences for the mother and the baby result from pre-eclampsia and eclampsia. These are associated with vasospasm, pathologic vascular lesions in multiple organ systems, increased platelet activation and subsequent activation of the coagulation system in the micro-vasculature[13]. Eclampsia is usually a consequence of pre-eclampsia consisting of central nervous system seizures, which often leave the patient unconscious; if untreated it may lead to death. The long-term sequelae of both pre-eclampsia or eclampsia are not well evaluated, and the burden of HDP stems mainly from deaths.

Formulating estimates of the global incidence of pre-eclampsia and eclampsia is difficult because of heterogeneity in definitions, problems related to the measurement of blood pressure in pregnant women, and the validity of urinary protein measurements in the diagnosis of pre-eclampsia.

However, recent estimates developed by WHO are built on somewhat stronger foundations than those for other direct obstetric complications described here. This is because WHO's Department of Reproductive Health and Research is currently undertaking a systematic review of pre-eclampsia and eclampsia. This has focused on recent, population-based studies from both developed and developing countries whose investigators made efforts to control and/or assure the diagnosis of pre-eclampsia and eclampsia (blood pressure and proteinuria measurements, documentation of seizure, *etc.*).

Based on initial results, the incidence of pre-eclampsia is estimated at 3.2% of live births, giving a total number of over 4 million cases each year, of which over 72,000 were fatal.

Obstructed labour

Labour is considered obstructed when the presenting part of the fetus cannot progress into the birth canal, despite strong uterine contractions. The most frequent cause of obstructed labour is cephalo-pelvic disproportion—a mismatch between the fetal head and the mother's pelvic brim. The fetus may be large in relation to the maternal pelvic brim, such as the fetus of a diabetic woman, or the pelvis may be contracted, which is more common when malnutrition is prevalent. Other causes of obstructed labour may be malpresentation or malposition of the fetus (shoulder, brow or occipito-posterior positions). In rare cases, locked twins or pelvic tumours can cause obstruction.

Neglected obstructed labour is a major cause of both maternal and newborn morbidity and mortality. The obstruction can only be alleviated by means of an operative delivery, either caesarean section or other instrumental delivery (forceps, vacuum extraction or simphysiotomy). Maternal complications include intrauterine infections following prolonged rupture of membranes, trauma to the bladder and/or rectum due to pressure from the fetal head or damage during delivery and ruptured uterus with consequent haemorrhage, shock or even death. Trauma to the bladder during vaginal or instrumental delivery may lead to stress incontinence.

By far the most severe and distressing long-term condition following obstructed labour is obstetric fistula—a hole which forms in the vaginal wall communicating into the bladder (vesico-vaginal fistula) or the rectum (recto-vaginal fistula) or both. In developing countries, fistulae are commonly the result of prolonged obstructed labour and follow pressure necrosis caused by impaction of the presenting part during difficult labour. In the infant, neglected obstructed labour may cause asphyxia leading to stillbirth, brain damage or neonatal death. Estimating the global dimensions of mortality and morbidity due to obstructed labour is difficult because of the absence of a clear definition and confusion of terms used by different practitioners[14]. The term 'dystocia' is most frequently used as an equivalent for obstructed labour, but it covers a broad range of conditions, from labour lasting more than 12 h to uterine rupture, feto-pelvic disproportion or abnormal fetal presentation. Moreover, estimating the duration of labour may be difficult, especially in settings without appropriate monitoring technology. It is, however, accepted that if obstruction cannot be overcome by manipulation or instrumental delivery, caesarean section is needed and thus it is possible to use the rate of caesarean section carried out for dystocia and mal-presentation as a proxy for the incidence of obstructed labour for regions where intervention is universally accessible. In settings where access to caesarean section is limited, obstructed labour is managed by means of instrumental deliveries. We assumed that in 90% of cases of obstructed labour, a caesarean section is carried out, and in the remaining 10% an instrumental delivery.

Based on extensive literature review and expert consensus, we estimate that obstructed labour occurs in around 4.6% of live births, giving a total number of cases of obstructed labour of over 6 million. Over 40,000 women die following neglected obstructed labour and some 73,000 suffer the most serious and debilitating non-fatal health outcome, obstetric fistula.

Abortion

The term 'abortion' covers a variety of conditions arising during early pregnancy, from ectopic pregnancy and hydatiform mole, through to spontaneous and induced abortion. There are important differences in the dimensions and nature of deaths and disabilities resulting from different kinds of abortion[15]. The overwhelming majority of deaths and disabilities caused by pregnancies with abortive outcome arise from the complications of unsafe abortion, defined as an abortion taking place outwith a health facility (or other place recognized by law) and/or provided by an unskilled person[16].

Unsafe abortion may lead to haemorrhage, infection and death, particularly in settings where there is poor access to hospital and medical care. When infection spreads upwards through the genital tract, causing damage to the fallopian tubes and ovaries, then pelvic inflammatory disease will develop. This condition causes pain and discomfort, and if left untreated, it can result in chronic pelvic pain, bilateral tubal occlusion (due to adhesions and scars formed around the uterus), and secondary infertility[17]. Secondary infertility is defined as failure to conceive again after an established pregnancy.

In countries where induced abortion is restricted and inaccessible, or even where abortion is legal but difficult to obtain, little information is available on abortion practice. Because of the difficulty of quantifying and classifying abortion in such circumstances, its occurrence tends to be unreported or under-reported. Surveys show that under-reporting[18–22] occurs where abortion is legal, and when taking place in clandestine conditions it may not be reported at all or as a spontaneous abortion (miscarriage). Estimates have to rely on adjustments to correct for misreporting and under-reporting, the degree of adjustment depending largely on which methods are commonly used to carry out the abortion, and assumptions of its relative incidence in rural and urban areas.

Data on incidence of unsafe abortion are tabulated in a database maintained by the Department of Reproductive Health and Research (RHR) in WHO. Reports included in the database are identified through a search of library databases and by tracing references. A recent in-depth review estimated a global incidence of unsafe abortion of over 14 unsafe abortions for every 100 live births, amounting to 68,000 abortion-related maternal deaths each year.

The views expressed in this article are those of the author and should not be taken to represent those of the World Health Organization.

References

1   World Health Organization. *International Statistical Classification of Diseases and Related Health Problems*, Tenth Revision. Geneva: WHO, 1992
2   Koonin LM *et al.* Maternal mortality surveillance, United States, 1980–1985. *Morb Mortal Wkly Rep* 1988; **37**: 19–29
3   Bouvier-Colle M-H *et al.* Reasons for the underreporting of maternal mortality in France, as indicated by a survey of all deaths of women of childbearing age. *Int J Epidemiol* 1991; **20**: 717–21
4   Atrash H, Alexander S, Berg C. Maternal mortality in developed countries: Not just a concern of the past. *Obstet Gynecol* 1995; **86**: 700–5
5   Lewis G, Drife J. *Why Mothers Die: The Confidential Enquiries into Maternal Deaths in the United Kingdom.* London: Royal College of Obstetricians and Gynaecologists, 2001
6   Chavkin W, Allen M. Questionable category of non-maternal deaths. *Am J Obstet Gynecol* 1993; **168**: 1640–1
7   Fortney JA *et al. Causes of death to women of reproductive age in Egypt.* Michigan State University Working Paper No. 49. Michigan State University, 1984
8   WHO, UNICEF, UNFPA. *Maternal Mortality in 2000: Estimates Developed by WHO, UNICEF and UNFPA.* Geneva: WHO, 2003
9   Fortney JA, Smith JB. Measuring maternal morbidity. In: Berer M, Ravindran TKS (eds) *Safe Motherhood Initiatives: Critical Issues. Reproductive Health Matters.* Blackwell Science, 1999
10 Abouzahr C. Antepartum and postpartum haemorrhage. In: Murray CJL, Lopez AD (eds) *Health Dimensions of Sex and Reproduction: the Global Burden of Sexually Transmitted Diseases, Maternal Conditions, Perinatal Disorders, and Congenital Anomalies.* Geneva: WHO, 1998
11 Adriaanse AH, Pel M, Bleker OP. Semmelweis: the combat against puerperal fever. *Eur J Obstet Gynecol Reprod Biol* 2000; **90**: 153–8

12 Abouzahr C, Aahman E, Guidotti R. Puerperal sepsis and other puerperal infections. In: Murray CJL, Lopez AD (eds) *Health Dimensions of Sex and Reproduction: The Global Burden of Sexually Transmitted Diseases, Maternal Conditions, Perinatal Disorders, and Congenital Anomalies.* Geneva: WHO, 1998

13 AbouZahr C, Guidotti R. Hypertensive disorders of pregnancy. In: Murray CJL, Lopez AD (eds) *Health Dimensions of Sex and Reproduction: The Global Burden of Sexually Transmitted Diseases, Maternal Conditions, Perinatal Disorders, and Congenital Anomalies.* Geneva: WHO, 1998

14 Ould El Joud D, Bouvier-Colle M-H, MOMA Group. Dystocia: study of its frequency and risk factors in seven cities in west Africa. *Int J Gynaecol Obstet* 2001; **74**: 171–8

15 Abouzahr C, Aahman E. Unsafe abortion and ectopic pregnancy. In: Murray CJL, Lopez AD (eds) *Health Dimensions of Sex and Reproduction: The Global Burden of Sexually Transmitted Diseases, Maternal Conditions, Perinatal Disorders, and Congenital Anomalies.* Geneva: WHO, 1998

16 *The Prevention and Management of Unsafe Abortion.* Report of a Technical Working Group, WHO/MSM/92.5. Geneva: WHO, 1992

17 Abouzahr C, Aaahman E, Guidotti R. Puerperal sepsis and other puerperal infections. In: Murray CJL, Lopez AD (eds) *Health Dimensions of Sex and Reproduction: The Global Burden of Sexually Transmitted Diseases, Maternal Conditions, Perinatal Disorders, and Congenital Anomalies.* Geneva: WHO, 1998

18 Wilcox AJ, Horney LF. Accuracy of spontaneous abortion recall. *Am J Epidemiol* 1984; **120**: 727–33

19 Jones EF, Forrest JD. Under-reporting of abortion in surveys of U.S. women: 1976 to 1988. *Demography* 1992; **29**: 113–26

20 van der Tak J. *Abortion, Fertility and Changing Legislation: An International Review.* Lexington: Lexington Books, 1974

21 Canto de Cetina TE *et al.* Aborto incompleto: caracteristicas de las pacientes tratadas en el Hospital O'Horan de Merida, Yucatan. *Salud pública de México* 1985; **27**: 507–13

22 Figa-Talamanca I *et al.* Illegal abortion: an attempt to assess its costs to the health services and its incidence in the community. *Int J Health Serv* 1986; **16**: 375–89

Safe Motherhood: a brief history of the global movement 1947–2002

Carla AbouZahr

World Health Organization, Geneva, Switzerland

The health of mothers has long been acknowledged to be a cornerstone of public health and attention to unacceptably high level of maternal mortality has been a feature of global health and development discussions since the 1980s. However, although a few countries have made remarkable progress in recent years, the reality has not generally followed the rhetoric. Health and development partners have failed to invest seriously in safe motherhood and examples of large-scale and sustained programmes are rare. Safe motherhood has tended to be seen as a subset of other programmes such as child survival or reproductive health and is often perceived to be too complex or costly for under-resourced and overstretched health care systems that have limited capacity. Despite this, a consensus has emerged about the interventions needed to reduce maternal mortality and there are good examples (historical and contemporary) of what can be achieved within a relatively short time period. The activities of both grassroots organizations and international health and development agencies have helped to build political will and momentum. Further progress in improving maternal health will require outspoken and determined champions from within the health system and the medical community, particularly the obstetricians and gynaecologists, and from among decision-makers and politicians. But in addition, substantial and long-term funding—by governments and by donor agencies—is an essential and still missing component.

*Correspondence to:
Carla AbouZahr,
Coordinator, Advocacy,
Communications and
Evaluation, Office of the
Executive Director,
Family and Community
Health, World Health
Organization,
20 Avenue Appia,
CH-1211 Geneva 27,
Switzerland.
E-mail:
abouzahrc@who.int*

Introduction

In the USA in 1900, there were about 700 maternal deaths for every 100,000 births, the same order of magnitude as in many developing countries today. One hundred years later, maternal mortality had fallen to less than 10 maternal deaths per 100,000 births. Similar precipitous declines occurred in other industrialized countries; in Sweden, the decline started well before 1900. By 1950, levels all over the developed world had coalesced at levels well below 100 per 100,000.

How did this change come about? The advent of technologies and drugs to prevent and manage obstetric complications was an important factor.

But by itself, this was not enough. Change came about at different times and rates in different countries, despite the general availability of the new technologies[1]. What made a difference was the political will to put the technologies into effect and this required two enabling conditions: the societal recognition that female social, economic and political emancipation was a prerequisite for social development (and its corollary, social peace) and the involvement of medical professionals in promoting that emancipation[1,2].

In the UK, for example, concern among the medical profession about continuing high levels of maternal mortality resulted in the setting up of enquiries into the subject by the Ministry of Health in 1928. These enquiries continued and were eventually turned into the ongoing Confidential Enquiries into Maternal Deaths. During the same period, government committees of enquiry were set up to 'investigate the general conditions of health among women … in view of indications that ill-health is more widespread and more serious than generally known'[3]. Representatives of women's organizations were included in the Committee 'on an entirely non-political basis'. This combination of the energies of the women's movement and senior medical professionals ensured that no government could afford to ignore women's health, particularly during pregnancy and childbirth.

There are important lessons to be learned from these experiences as we examine the short history of the global safe motherhood movement over the past half-century.

WHO, primary health care (PHC) and maternal and child health/family planning (MCH/FP)

Attention to the health of mothers and children is an explicit element of the WHO Constitution. Efforts '…to promote maternal and child health and welfare…' are included among the functions of the Organization. However, global interest in safe motherhood predates WHO's establishment. The League of Nations Health Section noted concerns about maternal mortality in 1930, reflecting the increasing interest in the topic in industrialized countries and the desire of many colonial powers to transfer to their colonies the benefits of medical progress that were by now so apparent.

It soon became clear that the simple transfer of medical care models from industrialized countries to developing ones was not going to work. This was the premise underlying the 1978 International Conference on Primary Health Care sponsored by WHO and UNICEF in Alma Ata. Countries made an explicit commitment to develop comprehensive health strategies that went beyond just providing services but that also addressed the underlying social, economic and political causes of ill-health.

Primary health care (PHC) would be universal, would address the needs of the poor, would encourage community participation and would focus on the main problems in the community, including maternal and child health care.

PHC fell victim to economics and was compromised by the adoption of selective interventions that attempted to bring technological fixes to health problems without addressing the underlying imbalances that create the problems in the first place[4]. This resulted in the implementation of vertical programmes whose outcomes could be readily measured, such as childhood immunization or growth monitoring. During the same period, concern about burgeoning populations (particularly in the developing world and among the poor) coincided with the development of new technologies for reducing fertility (contraceptive pills, IUDs and long-acting hormonal methods) and resulted in a major global effort to reduce levels of fertility in the developing world.

Population policies in developing countries were supported by UN agencies and a variety of non-governmental organizations (NGOs). Donors, anxious to demonstrate that their aid money was being well spent and in a drive for efficiency and effectiveness, often supported the establishment of free-standing 'vertical' family planning bodies, generally quite separate from other related government sectors such as health. In the meantime, other aspects of women's health, such as safety during pregnancy and childbirth, were neglected.

Where is the M?

During the 1970s and 1980s, advances in statistical techniques and the availability of data from household surveys and censuses resulted in increasing availability and reliability of data on infant mortality. But there had been no equivalent breakthroughs with regard to the measurement of maternal mortality, the dimensions of which remained largely hidden. During 1985, WHO, with funding from UNFPA, provided support to the first community studies on levels of maternal mortality in developing countries[5]. Based on these studies, and what little information was available from vital registration and hospital studies, WHO produced the first 'guestimates' of the extent of the problem and announced that half a million maternal deaths were occurring each year, 99% of them in developing countries. By 1987, Dr Hafdan Mahler, then the WHO's Director-General, was able to assert that 'Sound estimates based on new data are ... the foundation of our current understanding and concern'[6].

In February that year, WHO, UNFPA and the World Bank jointly sponsored the first international Safe Motherhood Conference in Nairobi.

The conference declared that '…something can, should—indeed must—be done, starting with the commitment of heads of states and governments'[6]. The Conference was the effective starting point of what came to be known as the Safe Motherhood Initiative (SMI). The three original co-sponsors were later joined in the SMI Inter-Agency Group (IAG) by UNDP, UNICEF, IPPF and The Population Council with Family Care International (FCI) serving as an informal secretariat.

A key perception to emerge over this period was the relative neglect of women's health compared with the attention then being given to child survival and health, a point most forcefully made by Allan Rosenfield and Deborah Maine in their seminal article 'Where is the M in MCH?'[7].

A by-product of child survival?

Two years after Nairobi, the World Summit for Children took place in New York in 1989. In contrast to the Safe Motherhood Conference, the Children's Summit was attended by heads of state, executive heads of UN agencies, and senior representatives of countries, NGOs and the international development community. The Child Summit included reduction in maternal mortality as one of the goals to be monitored along with increases in antenatal care attendance. However, maternal mortality was viewed almost entirely within the context of ensuring the survival and health of children. As the Executive Director of UNICEF, James Grant, noted, '…the emphasis on goals for maternal mortality is largely a by-product of child survival efforts'[8].

Where is the W?

The failure to address maternal health as a good thing, in and of itself, independent of its impact on child health, did not pass unnoticed among women's health advocates. The United Nations Decade for Women, 1976–1985, had helped focus attention on women's rights and health. The Decade culminated in the formulation of the 'Forward Looking Strategies' which called for a reduction in maternal mortality by the year 2000. Women's health advocates stressed the importance of women's health in its own right and were suspicious of any hint that women's interests might be subsumed to those of their infants.

The Women's Global Network for Reproductive Rights and the Latin American & Caribbean Women's Health Network/ISIS International, issued a Call to Action on 28 May 1990, declared International Day of Action for Women's Health[9]. This campaign was instrumental in drawing attention to the issue of maternal mortality, particularly in Latin America.

The campaign focused particular attention on unsafe abortion and on the poor quality of care meted out to women (particularly poor or indigenous women) by the formal health care system. Maternal mortality was presented as a political challenge with responsibility firmly attributed to high level decision-makers: 'To cure the health problems of women is to acknowledge that oppression—and health problems—are not determined by biology but by a social system based on the power of sex and class'[10].

By the early 1990s, NGOs around the world were working in the area of safe motherhood, often at a very local level, engaging in community-based research, participating in awareness-raising or public education campaigns, promoting workshops, meetings or media events and even delivering care[11].

From MCH/FP to reproductive health

During the mid-1990s, a series of international conferences, organized under the auspices of the United Nations, led to significant re-evaluation of development efforts. At the International Conference on Population and Development (ICPD) in Cairo in 1994, the Fourth World Conference for Women (FWCW) in Beijing in 1995, and the Social Summit in Copenhagen in 1995, attention was focused again on the social, cultural and gender-based determinants of health and development. Safe motherhood was now viewed within a more comprehensive reproductive or women's health context.

At the same time, a wide-ranging, grassroots movement expressed opposition to the prevailing dominance of demographically driven family planning programmes. These developments signalled a broadening of the women's health agenda to address previously neglected problems such as female genital mutilation, violence and trafficking. Also by now, the global impact of the HIV epidemic was undeniable, as was its devastating impact on women and children and its fundamental gender dimensions. No longer the 'gay disease', HIV was seen to both reflect, and to exacerbate, social inequalities and vulnerabilities. In sub-Saharan Africa above all, and in all settings with generalized epidemics, HIV is a gender issue. Women are more likely to be infected than men, they become infected at younger ages, and they bear, more heavily than do men, the social and economic consequences of illness.

The A-word

The expansion of the women's health and development agenda had some unintended, and perverse, consequences for safe motherhood. Among some women's health activists, ambivalence about safe motherhood strengthened. Was safe motherhood really about women's rights and health or was it just a matter of 'motherhood and apple pie'? Even the name seemed to draw attention to the outcome of the pregnancy rather than to the choice to become pregnant in the first place.

The women's movement recognized early on that abortion would be the most contentious aspect of efforts to reduce maternal mortality. Almost universally, they identified societal reluctance to endorse the right of women to decide whether and when to have children and to provide both contraceptive and abortion services to enable them to do so safely. This seriously complicated efforts to draw attention to safe motherhood. Among anti-abortionists, safe motherhood was seen as the Trojan horse for the introduction of legal abortion. Funders interested in supporting safe motherhood programmes became wary and today certain donors cannot be approached for support to projects or programmes that include an abortion-related component.

Problems such as these have added to the ambivalence and hesitation of policy-makers. In some countries, for example, although national plans for the reduction in maternal mortality exist, government officials have an ambivalent attitude towards reproductive health which has hampered implementation[12].

Safe motherhood is a human right

Despite these developments, the combination of the paradigm shifts that happened in Cairo and Beijing, and the reaffirmation of the health and human rights linkages, brought a powerful new dimension to support for safe motherhood. Maternal deaths, it was argued, are unlike other deaths. Pregnancy is not a disease but a normal physiological process that women must engage in for the sake of humanity[13]. Whereas the elimination or eradication of disease is a rational and laudable endeavour, the same strategy cannot be applied to maternal mortality. There is no pathogen to control, no vector to eradicate. Women will continue to need care during pregnancy and childbirth as long as humanity continues to reproduce itself. Failure to take action to prevent maternal death amounts to discrimination because only women face the risk.

This perception of the different nature of maternal mortality within the general context of illness and disease has stimulated renewed interest in a rights-based approach to safe motherhood. Defining maternal death as a 'social injustice' as well as a 'health disadvantage' obligates governments to address the causes of poor maternal health through their political, health and legal systems. This raises the option of using international treaties and national constitutions that address basic human rights to advocate for safe motherhood and to hold governments accountable for their actions—or inaction[14].

World Health Day 1998

The burgeoning interest in reproductive health and rights during the late 1990s gave further impetus to efforts to keep safe motherhood high on the international health agenda. In 1996, the SMI Inter-Agency Group embarked upon a 2 year effort to bring maternal health to a wider audience and to a higher level of decision-makers. The preparatory phase culminated in an international technical consultation in Colombo, Sri Lanka, in October 1997[15]. The consultation brought together safe motherhood specialists, programme planners and decision-makers from international and national agencies. The discussions at Colombo helped to forge greater consensus on the interventions needed to reduce maternal mortality.

WHO determined that World Health Day 1998 would be devoted to safe motherhood, with the slogan 'Pregnancy is special: let's make it safe'. Around the world, street parties, theatrical presentations, marches, media events and poster campaigns focused on safe motherhood. In Washington, DC, USA, executive heads of major international agencies came together with high level politicians from the developing world and the USA first lady to issue a Call to Action for safe motherhood.

The Call to Action represented a significant upgrading of efforts for maternal health. Since then, new entrants to the safe motherhood field have come to add their weight to the growing movement, including the White Ribbon Alliance for Safe Motherhood, and Safe Motherhood Initiatives USA. Others, already involved in safe motherhood, such as Columbia University, PATH, AVSC International and Marie Stopes International have increased their existing commitment. UN agencies have promised greater resources and visibility, for example, through WHO's Making Pregnancy Safer Initiative, UNICEF's Women-Friendly Health Services strategy, UNFPA's Programme Advisory Note for Reducing Maternal Mortality and Morbidity, and The World Bank's Safe Motherhood Action Plan. Four agencies—WHO, UNFPA, UNICEF and the World Bank—issued a joint statement on the essential strategies needed to reduce maternal mortality and affirming their collective engagement in support of safe motherhood[16].

A professional responsibility

As the international interest in maternal health has grown, so has the commitment of those health care professionals closest to the problem—midwives, nurses and obstetricians. Of all the allies that safe motherhood needs, none is as crucial as the medical community. It was, after all, the alliance of medical professionals with women's advocates that forged the strong links needed to ensure government commitment to reduction in maternal mortality in the UK during the 1930s. On the international stage too, medical professional associations acknowledged their roles and responsibilities in safe motherhood early on. International Nurses Day 1988 was on the theme of safe motherhood. Since 1987, the International Confederation of Midwives has regularly organized precongress workshops on different aspects of safe motherhood midwifery before the triennial congresses. The 1990 precongress workshop was instrumental in opening up debate among midwifery associations about delegation of responsibility and the need for training of midwives to deal with emergency obstetric complications. Later workshops addressed issues of monitoring, quality, abortion and HIV/AIDS.

The WHO and the International Federation of Gynaecologists and Obstetricians (FIGO) Task Force was established in 1982 to draw attention to safe motherhood at both global and regional levels. Precongress workshops have tackled a range of reproductive health issues including safe motherhood. But the fine sentiments voiced at such meetings were rarely followed by practical action. A 1998 article in the *Lancet* took the profession to task for failing to assume its responsibilities and leaving Safe Motherhood 'an orphan initiative'[17].

It was not until 1997, however, that FIGO moved from words to specific action with the establishment of the FIGO Save the Mothers Fund, a north–south partnership to support direct training projects between ObGyn associations. In addition to support from UNFPA and the World Bank, the Fund receives funds from Pharmacia-Upjohn, a rare instance of private involvement in safe motherhood. This initiative is illustrative of the increasing role of the ObGyn which has grown with the emerging consensus that effectively addressing the challenge of maternal mortality implies doing something to ensure that all women with complications—whether emergency or not—can access the needed medical care.

At the same time, the medical profession has to contend with frank mistrust on the part of some women's advocacy groups who have sensed a tendency for doctors to overmedicalize a natural process, a diagnosis supported by the inexorably rising rates of caesarean delivery around the world.

The Millennium Declaration

The consensus on the need to reduce maternal mortality expressed at the international conferences of the 1990s laid the foundation for its inclusion among the health and development priorities that have emerged at the start of the new millennium. In December 2000, representatives of 189 countries collectively endorsed the Millennium Declaration, which explicitly calls for improvements in maternal health and reductions in levels of maternal mortality. This global commitment has been summarized in the Millennium Development Goals (MDGs), which have been commonly accepted as a framework for measuring development progress, focusing on efforts to achieve significant, measurable improvements in people's lives, especially for the poor[18].

The inclusion of maternal health as one of the eight MDGs, the unambiguous focus on a maternal mortality reduction target and the inclusion of a skilled attendant at delivery as an indicator of progress provide an unparalleled opportunity to re-energize safe motherhood efforts. The MDGs are being used to reorient the work of countries, programmes and agencies. Because the eight MDGs are mutually complementary and reinforcing, the opportunities for achieving sustainable progress are greater than they ever have been. In addition to the three goals that relate directly to health outcomes (maternal and child health and communicable diseases), other goals relate indirectly to health because they focus on important determinants—poverty, gender, education, water and sanitation. Thus, working cross-sectorally, with many partners and addressing systemic constraints to progress is the most effective way of achieving progress.

Safe motherhood needs a health system

One of the most problematic issues with which safe motherhood efforts have had to contend has been the preference of donor agencies for 'vertical' focused programmes, perceived (often correctly) to be more effective in reaching their target audiences and in delivering their promises. Such approaches have apparently achieved results in the area of child survival—why should they not do so for mothers too?

The answer is that they do not work when it comes to reducing maternal mortality. We know this because they have been tried and found wanting. In the early years of the Safe Motherhood Initiative, many programmes focused exclusively on a single component such as training traditional birth attendants or providing antenatal care. Only in 1997 at the Sri Lanka meeting did a consensus emerge that making motherhood safer required a full panoply of interventions, comprising health care for women throughout pregnancy and delivery and including access to skilled medical care for complications. The implications for health systems are significant. Implementing safe motherhood programmes requires that human resources are in place (trained, deployed and paid), that they have the necessary drugs, equipment and supplies, and that they are able to function in a supportive policy, regulatory and legal environment. Ironically, today there is a growing perception that vertical approaches are of limited effectiveness in dealing with childhood conditions too. And providing care and support to people living with HIV/AIDS faces similar requirements. The era of single interventions that bypass the health system appears to be well and truly over.

How much will it cost?

Establishing and maintaining functional health systems costs money and it is a common perception that safe motherhood programmes are so complex that poor countries simply cannot afford them. The historical evidence does not support this view however. In Sri Lanka, a country which achieved remarkable reductions in levels of maternal mortality during the second half of the 20th century, total expenditure on maternal health care (recurrent and capital expenditures) averages 0.23% of GDP, or around 12% of total government expenditure on health. Costs were higher at the beginning of the programme during the 1950s and gradually declined as a result of a combination of increased efficiency and the growth of the private sector[19]. In Malaysia, similar substantial declines in levels of maternal mortality were achieved while maintaining maternal health care expenditures at less than 0.4% of GDP[19].

WHO has developed a simple spreadsheet to assist in estimating the cost of implementing a set of safe motherhood interventions at the district level[20]. The model includes a standard set of assumptions representing a hypothetical rural district population. Using locally collected data, the model can be used to estimate the actual cost of current services, as well as the cost of upgrading the district health system to meet standards of care for the prevention and management of obstetric problems. Included are estimates of total, per capita and per-birth costs for the district. The estimates are further broken down by input (such as drugs, vaccines, salaries and infrastructure), by intervention (such as management of normal birth, haemorrhage, eclampsia and sepsis), and by service location or level (hospital, health centre and health post).

Follow the money

These examples notwithstanding, countries currently facing high levels of maternal mortality will need to find significant sums to put into place the essential health system requirements for safe motherhood. Such resources do not necessarily have to be found from external sources. A recent study comparing expenditures on various reproductive health services in Sri Lanka and Egypt[21] found that despite the very different health situations in the two countries, the overall pattern of costs was broadly similar. The authors concluded that although providing safe childbirth and routine obstetric and gynaecological services to women was the most expensive element of a package of reproductive health services, addressing inefficiencies in health systems would probably offer the most effective solution to the resources dilemma.

The same study also found, however, that the pattern of donor support does not reflect the actual resource requirements for different aspects of reproductive health, and that the provision of care during pregnancy and childbirth remains the neglected area despite all the commitments made at international fora. International funding is mostly targeted at family planning services, and gives minimal support to safe motherhood and inpatient services.

Better targeted and more generous external assistance will be vital if countries with high levels of maternal mortality are to be able to begin to make significant inroads into the problem. In 1987, WHO estimated that less than US$2 out of every US$10 of international resources devoted to health was spent on maternal-child health and family planning[22]. During the preparations for the 1994 Cairo conference, a similar exercise produced rather similar results[23] and more recent estimates have not led to a revision of the basic premise that insufficient funding is available for safe motherhood[24]. Few donor agencies are able to provide clear statements on support for safe motherhood. UNFPA categorizes population programmes and activities into broad groups, with safe motherhood activities grouped under 'basic reproductive health services given at primary health care level' along with training of traditional birth attendant (TBAs), antenatal care and eradicating female genital mutilation (NIDI 2000). Several major donors, USAID among them, do not have a separate budget for maternal health. Recent initiatives in donor funding and disbursement, such as SWAPS, encourage basket funding for a range of integrated programme activities and make it harder to track funds specifically allocated to safe motherhood.

Of the UN agencies, only the World Bank has carried out a systematic analysis of its funding for safe motherhood activities and is now the largest source of external assistance for safe motherhood. In recent years, the Bank has shifted its support from programmes focused almost entirely on child health or family planning activities to programmes comprising activities related to safe delivery and management of obstetric complications.

However, there are some encouraging signs on the resources front. The USAID-supported JHPIEGO Maternal and Neonatal Health project, established in 1999, has access to up to US$50 million over the first 5 years. Significant new funding for safe motherhood has been generated through Columbia University's Joseph L. Mailman School of Public Health with resources from the Bill and Melinda Gates Foundation. For example, UNFPA and Columbia University have signed a pact through which US$8 million will be allocated to improving the availability of emergency obstetric care in developing countries. The Gates Foundation has also provided significant support to the Aberdeen University Initiative for Maternal Mortality Programme Assessment (IMMPACT). On the other hand, WHO's Making Pregnancy Safer Initiative has a mere US$3 million from WHO's regular budget at its disposal for the current biennium (2000–2001) and it is anticipated that additional funds will need to be raised from voluntary contributions. With resources at these kinds of levels, progress towards safer motherhood will inevitably be limited.

Conclusions

The striking reductions in levels of maternal mortality observed in developed countries during the early part of the last century are attributable to the bringing together of technical requirements (data systems, professional expertise and access to technologies) with political enabling conditions (awareness of the problem and commitment to act). Is such a combination of circumstances in place today in the developing world? Certainly the technologies are available and cost-effective. The political will exists, as manifested by the Millennium Declaration, which was endorsed at the highest levels by all countries. Health care professionals and women's advocates espouse the cause of safe motherhood. Perhaps the missing element is health sector readiness—the combination of financial, human and organizational resources that is needed to provide services required to the people who need them. Both recipient countries and donors will need to invest in this area if the political will that now exists to tackle maternal mortality is to be translated into action.

The views expressed in this article are those of the author and should not be taken to represent those of the World Health Organization.

References

1   De Brouwere V, Tonglet R, Van Lerberghe W. La 'Maternité sans risque' dans les pays en développement: les lecons de l'histoire. *Studies in Health Services Organization and Policy*, 1997, 6. Antwerp, Belgium: ITG Press
2   Van Lerberghe W, De Brouwere V. Of blind alleys and things that have worked: history's lessons on reducing maternal mortality. In: de Brouwere V, Van Lerberghe W (eds) *Safe Motherhood Strategies: A Review of the Evidence. Studies in Health Services Organisation and Policy*, 2001, 17. Antwerp, Belgium: ITG Press
3   Spring-Rice M. *Working-class Wives: Their Health and Conditions*. London: Pelican Books, 1939
4   Werner D, Saunders D. *Questioning the Solution: the Politics of Primary Health Care and Child Survival*. Palo Alto, CA: HealthWrights, 1997
5   WHO. *Prevention of Maternal Mortality: Report of the WHO Interregional Meeting, November 1985*. WHO/FHE/86.1. Geneva: World Health Organization, 1986

6   Mahler H. *Address to the Nairobi Safe Motherhood Conference.* Geneva: World Health Organization, 1987

7   Rosenfield A, Maine D. Maternal mortality—a neglected tragedy. Where is the M in MCH? *Lancet* 1985; **2**: 83–5

8   Grant J. Statement to the Fourth International Child Survival Conference, March 1–3 1990, Bangkok, Thailand

9   *Maternal Mortality and Morbidity: A Call to Women for Action.* Amsterdam: Women's Global Network for Reproductive Rights and the Latin American & Caribbean Women's Health Network/ISIS International, 1990

10 Araujo and Diniz. The campaign in Brazil: From the technical to the political. In: *Maternal Mortality and Morbidity: A Call to Women for Action.* Amsterdam: Women's Global Network for Reproductive Rights and the Latin American & Caribbean Women's Health Network/ISIS International, 1990

11 WHO. *Women's Groups, NGOs and Safe Motherhood* (doc.WHO/FHE/MSM/92.3). Geneva: World Health Organization, 1992

12 UNFPA. Safe motherhood evaluation. *Evaluation Findings.* Office of Oversight and Evaluation, *Evaluation Findings*, issue 10, January 1999. New York: UNFPA.

13 Fathalla M. *From Obstetrics and Gynaecology to Women's Health: The Road Ahead.* New York, London: Parthenon Publishing, 1997

14 Cook R. Advance safe motherhood through human rights. In: Starrs A (ed) *The Safe Motherhood Action Agenda: Priorities for the Next Decade.* New York: Family Care International, 1997

15 *Report on the safe motherhood technical consultation* (18–23 October 1997, Colombo, Sri Lanka). Final report on the program to mark the tenth anniversary of the Safe Motherhood Initiative. Safe Motherhood Inter-Agency Group, 1999. New York: Family Care International.

16 WHO/UNFPA/UNICEF/World Bank. *Reduction of Maternal Mortality: A Joint WHO/UNFPA/UNICEF/World Bank Statement.* Geneva: World Health Organization, 1999

17 Weil O, Fernandez H. Is safe motherhood an orphan initiative? *Lancet* 1999; **354**: 940–3

18 Fifty-fifth session of the United Nations General Assembly, item 40 of the provisional agenda. Follow-up to the outcome of the Millennium Summit. *Road Map Towards the Implementation of the United Nations Millennium Declaration*, Report of the Secretary-General (A/56/326). September 2001

19 Pathmanathan I *et al. Investing in Maternal Health: Learning from Malaysia and Sri Lanka.* Washington, DC: The World Bank, Human Development Network, 2003

20 WHO. The *Mother-Baby Package Costing Spreadsheet.* WHO/FCH/RHR/99.17. Geneva: WHO, 1999

21 Rannan-Eliya RP, Berman P, Eltigani EE, de Silva I, Somanathan A, Sumathiratne V. *Expenditures for Reproductive Health Services in Egypt and Sri Lanka.* Occasional Paper 13. Sri Lanka: Institute of Policy Studies of Sri Lanka, 2000

22 WHO. Safe motherhood factsheet prepared for the Nairobi Conference. WHO, 1987

23 SIDA. *Population Policies Reconsidered.* Monograph. Stockholm, SIDA: 1993

24 United Nations Population Division. Commission on Population and Development. Report of the Secretary-General on the flow of financial resources for assisting in the implementation of the Programme of Action of the International Conference on Population and Development E/CN.9/2002/4. New York: United Nations, 2002

Beyond the Numbers: reviewing maternal deaths and complications to make pregnancy safer

Gwyneth Lewis

Department of Reproductive Health and Research, World Health Organization, Geneva, Switzerland

'Whose faces are behind the numbers? What were their stories? What were their dreams? They left behind children and families. They also left behind clues as to why their lives end so early[1]'

Avoiding maternal deaths is possible, even in resource-poor countries, but requires the right kind of information on which to base programmes. Knowing the level of maternal mortality is not enough; we need to understand the underlying factors that led to the deaths. Each maternal death or case of life-threatening complication has a story to tell and can provide indications on practical ways of addressing its causes and determinants. Maternal death or morbidity reviews provide evidence of where the main problems in overcoming maternal mortality and morbidity may lie, produce an analysis of what can be done in practical terms and highlight the key areas requiring recommendations for health sector and community action as well as guidelines for improving clinical outcomes. The information gained from such enquiries must be used as a prerequisite for action.

'A pregnant woman has one foot in the grave'

*Correspondence to:
Gwyneth Lewis, Director
and editor of the United
Kingdom Confidential
Enquiries into Maternal
Deaths and member of
the Making Pregnancy
Safer Team, Department
of Reproductive Health
and Research, World
Health Organization, 20
Avenue Appia, CH-1211
Geneva 27, Switzerland.
E-mail: Gwyneth.Lewis@
doh.gsi.gov.uk*

This traditional African saying summarizes the difficulties faced by pregnant women in many parts of the world. As discussed in Chapter 1, which provides a résumé of the global burden of maternal deaths and disability, each year throughout the world approximately eight million women are suffering pregnancy-related complications and over half a million will die[2]. In some developing countries, one in 11 pregnant women may die of pregnancy-related complications compared to one in 5000–10,000 in some developed countries.

The most recent world estimate of the overall maternal mortality ratio (MMR) is around 400 per 100,000 live births. By the Regions of the World Health Organization (WHO), the MMR is highest in Africa (830), followed by Asia (330), Oceania, excluding Japan, Australia and New Zealand

(240), Latin America and the Caribbean (190), and the developed countries (20). These figures hide wide inter-country variations and even within countries major discrepancies exist between the rich and poor and urban and remote areas. With the exception of Afghanistan and Haiti, all other of the 22 countries with MMRs in excess of 1000 per 100,000 live births are in sub-Saharan Africa.

These figures represent the largest public health discrepancy in the world. Each death or long-term complication represents an individual tragedy for the woman, her partner, her children and family. More tragically, most deaths are avoidable. It is estimated that more than 80% of maternal deaths could be prevented or avoided through actions that are proven to be effective and affordable, even in resource-poor countries[3]. For example, reviews such as have occurred in Egypt[4] and elsewhere have shown that the quality of care provided to the women is a key determinant in maternal outcome and that, sometimes, simple changes in practice can save many lives.

Why do mothers really die?

While it may appear simple to use MMRs for purposes of comparison or for tracking change over time or to analyse what vital statistics may be available to attribute the causes of death to clinical categories, neither method provides any information on the real and underlying reasons why women die.

MMRs give no indication of either from what clinical conditions women are dying, what factors led to their deaths or whether the majority of deaths occur amongst women from any particular groups in society or geographical areas. And MMRs cannot be used to determine the estimates of pregnancy-related complications which the women have survived but have resulted in long-term severe disabilities. In the UK, the apparently low MMR hides a 20-fold difference in maternal mortality amongst women from the most vulnerable groups in society compared to those from the most affluent[5]. These women died from a wide variety of causes and it was only when their deaths were assessed by the UK Confidential Enquiry into Maternal Deaths (UKCEMD) that the commonest factor, lack of regular contact with the health services, was identified. Overcoming these inequalities in access to health care will be the cornerstone of the forthcoming National Service Framework for Maternity and Children's Health in England.

Death certificates, where they exist, and even if the coding of cause of death is correct, also give no information on the real reasons why the women died. The main direct clinical causes of maternal death are listed in vital statistic data as haemorrhage, sepsis, eclampsia, obstructed labour and unsafe abortion. But these numbers still hide the real reason why these women may be dying. For example a woman dying from haemorrhage may have not understood the need to seek care, may not have had money or access to transport, may have been deterred from seeking help by inappropriate traditional practices, may have received inadequate clinical care or may have been treated in a facility without access to blood products. Knowing the precise reasons why such women die will enable a start to be made in addressing the specific problems to be overcome. These may include community and personal awareness, the provision of transport, updating health care worker training or improving the blood supply.

The reality is that the vast majority of women die usually because they do not receive the health care that they need. This may be the result of a lack of basic health care provision or through, for whatever reason, an inability to access the local health care services. As discussed in Chapter 4 on skilled care, only 53% of women in developing countries receive assistance from a skilled attendant at birth. Some women are denied access to care because of cultural beliefs and practices, seclusion or because responsibility for decision making falls to her husband or other family members. In many cases, the failure of support for pregnant women by families, partners or their government reflects the societal value placed on women's lives.

Maternal complications and disability

Maternal deaths are the tip of the iceberg of maternal disability and for every woman who dies, many more will survive but often suffer from life long disabilities. These are not only personal and family tragedies, for example as described in Chapter 15 on obstructed labour and obstetric fistula, but their loss of the ability to work or support the family also carries a huge economic burden. Chapter 1 has described the inherent difficulties in trying to estimate the number of severe maternal morbidities. A conservative estimate of 20 disabilities per maternal death made by the WHO AFRO Region was used for a recent economic impact study. The results of this suggested that, unless women's health care provision improved, the economic burden from maternal deaths and disabilities in Africa alone would lead to a $45 billion loss in productivity over the next 10 years[4].

It is difficult to determine accurately the precise number of women suffering from morbidity for many reasons, not least the fact that in many parts of the world the woman will never have had contact with the health services. However, in the developed world, a number of studies have been published on the incidence of severe maternal morbidity, or 'near-misses', but comparison between them is difficult because of the different definitions of morbidity used. The death to near-miss ratio in these studies ranges from 1:5[6] to 1:118[7] per maternal death. But whatever the death to disability ratio actually is, the fact is that, as with the MMR, it will always be too high. Since women are disabled by the same conditions that cause maternal deaths, reducing the risk factors for maternal deaths will also reduce the numbers of women who experience significant medical or psychological problems before, during or after birth, sometimes with long-lasting or permanent sequelae.

Looking beyond the numbers

Whilst the numbers of maternal deaths and severe complaints are stark, they tell only part of the story. In particular, they tell us nothing about the *faces behind the numbers*, the individual stories of suffering and distress and the real underlying reasons why particular women died. Most of all, they tell us nothing about why women continue to die in a world where the knowledge and resources to prevent such deaths are available or attainable. While it is important to keep monitoring overall levels of maternal mortality at global, regional and national levels, for both identification and advocacy purposes, statistics about the level of maternal mortality do not help us identify what can be done to prevent or avoid such unnecessary deaths.

Today, with better understanding of the difficulties involved in measuring levels of maternal mortality, and the cost of conducting a full-scale exercise to determine overall MMRs, there is increasing interest in directing a larger share of limited resources into efforts to understand why the problem persists and what can be done to avert maternal deaths and cases of severe morbidity. Answering these questions is vital for programme planners, managers and service providers. In order to help address this, the WHO's Making Pregnancy Safer initiative will shortly publish 'Beyond the Numbers'[8], a guide which describes a number of strategies and approaches to review cases of maternal death or disability to help understand why mothers really die to enable the necessary actions to be taken on the results.

'Beyond the Numbers': a new approach to diagnosis

The methodologies for understanding why women die or suffer long-term complications, described in 'Beyond the Numbers', are designed to be a first step in the process of planning, implementing and evaluating strategies to helping reduce maternal deaths and disability. As with any life-threatening clinical condition, a diagnosis needs to be made before the appropriate treatment can be provided. It is this crucial first step that has often been lacking in the design of well-meaning but eventually partially ineffective programmes for maternal ill-health reduction. The use of these techniques can help with the diagnosis of the underlying causes, for example, are women dying because:

they were unaware of the need for care, or unaware of the warning signs of problems in pregnancy?

or

the services did not exist, or were inaccessible for other reasons such as distance, cost or sociocultural barriers?

or

are women dying because the care they receive in traditional or modern health services is inadequate or actually harmful?

Answering such questions and taking positive action on the results is often more important than knowing the precise level of magnitude of maternal mortality. The various approaches described in 'Beyond the Numbers' will enable, and empower, health professionals and authorities to act on the answers to these and other important questions about why women die during pregnancy and childbirth. In planning any such review, it is important to build in sustainability from the beginning so that such activities become a routine part of clinical practice and health information systems.

Maternal mortality and safe motherhood committees, as well as all other stakeholders in maternal health, for example international agencies, non-governmental organizations, community groups and health advocates, will also be able to use the information generated from using these approaches. The results of these reviews can have a powerful advocacy role and can also be used by politicians and those in other positions of influence to raise awareness and mobilize resources.

In the UK, the most dramatic decline in a local MMR was achieved in Rochdale, an industrial town in the poorest area of England, which, in 1928, had a MMR of over 900 per 100,000 live births, more than double the national average of the time. Following local concern, the local public health department undertook a confidential enquiry into maternal deaths in the community and associated hospitals, action on the results of which reduced the MMR to 280 per 100,000 pregnancies by 1934, the lowest in the country. This decline took only 6 years and this achievement was all the more remarkable as it took place during a time of severe economic depression. As the report states: 'it is important to note that the results were obtained by a change in spirit and method and without any alteration in the personnel or any substantial increase in public expenditure'[9]. The review ascertained that the leading causes of death—haemorrhage, eclampsia and sepsis—were compounded by the women's lack of knowledge about pregnancy and warning signs of complications and the far too frequent use of forceps and other techniques to deliver the women quickly. The local medical and midwifery profession worked together to introduce a public health education campaign, to reduce unnecessary obstetric practices and to introduce new standards of care. As the published report states 'all available agencies such as the platform, the pulpit, the factory supervisor, and the press, were used to awaken the community to the need for antenatal care and the signs and symptoms of complications'.

The above case history clearly demonstrates how generating information about the real reasons why mothers die can be used by health professionals, health care planners and managers to save women's lives. All the approaches described in 'Beyond the Numbers' go beyond counting the numbers of cases of death to understanding why they happened and how they can be prevented or avoided. The approaches can be adapted for use in any country and in any setting by anyone with a commitment to safe motherhood. Acting on the results of these studies offers an opportunity for all involved in planning and providing services for pregnant, delivering and recently delivered women to make a real and lasting difference to their lives and those of their families and communities. Depending on the results, and where the reviews took place, the outcomes may range from local to national public education campaigns, the mobilization of community resources, the restructuring of local clinics to make them more accessible or changing clinical practice by the development of local or national clinical guidelines. Experience from the use of these approaches has shown that although the initial implementation is often on a small scale by a few committed individuals, they can subsequently be implemented on a broader scale, including at the national level.

The five key approaches

'Beyond the Numbers' describes five different types of review or audit that can be used in a variety of settings, from the very simple to the sophisticated, to help reduce maternal deaths and disability. They can be used at different levels, from the national to local, and in communities, health facilities or both. Further, the approaches can be used for two specific health outcomes (maternal deaths and women who survive life-threatening complications) and for one kind of process (clinical care). These approaches are summarized in Table 1.

Whilst it is beyond the scope of this short chapter to describe each approach in detail, with its attendant pre-requisites, advantages and disadvantages,

'Beyond the Numbers' does just that. It contains a general overview, chapters on how to decide which approach may be best to adopt for a given situation or population, a general chapter on underlying principles common to each methodology and specific chapters for each technique. These specific chapters describe each methodology in detail, and the practical steps required to set up such a study as well as providing helpful case histories. The book is accompanied by a companion CD-ROM which contains practical examples of existing questionnaires that have been developed and used in undertaking such studies in a number of areas in the world. These are available for adaptation by others wishing to adopt similar methodologies. The information will also be available on the WHO RHR website in due course[11].

Deciding which of the approaches to use is influenced by two considerations, namely which level is appropriate for the review, and what kind of cases will be studied. In terms of level, there are essentially five options— the review can be conducted at the community, health care facility, or district, regional or national levels. In choosing which cases to study, a decision needs to be taken whether these will be outcomes or processes. Not all locations are suited to reviewing all types of cases. For example, auditing clinical practice, for resource-poor countries, may be more feasible at

Table 1 Summary of approaches described in 'Beyond the Numbers'

Approach	Definition
Community-based maternal death reviews (verbal autopsies)	A method of finding out the medical causes of death and ascertaining the personal, family or community factors that may have contributed to the deaths in women who died outside of a medical facility
Facility-based maternal deaths review	A qualitative, in-depth investigation of the causes of and circumstances surrounding maternal deaths occurring at health facilities. Deaths are initially identified at the facility level but such reviews may be expanded to identify the combination of factors at the facility and in the community that contributed to the death and which deaths were avoidable
Confidential enquiries into maternal deaths	A systematic multi-disciplinary anonymous investigation of all or a representative sample of maternal deaths occurring at an area, regional (state) or national level. It identifies the numbers, causes and avoidable or remediable factors associated with them
Reviews of severe morbidity (near misses)	The identification and assessment of cases in which pregnant women survive obstetric complications. These can be used in addition to reviewing maternal deaths through any of the other approaches described here
	There is no universally applicable definition for such cases and it is important that the definition used in any review be appropriate to local circumstances to enable local improvements in maternal care
Clinical audit	Clinical audit has been described as a quality improvement process that seeks to improve patient care and outcomes through systematic review of aspects of the structure, processes and outcomes of care against explicit criteria and the subsequent implementation of change. Where indicated, changes are implemented at an individual, team or service level and further monitoring is used to confirm improvement in healthcare delivery[10]

Table 2 Different approaches at different levels and for different topics

Level	Outcome		
	Maternal deaths	Severe complications	Clinical practice
Community	Verbal autopsy (community-based death reviews)	No	No
Facility or groups of facilities	Facility-based deaths review	Severe morbidity or 'near miss' case review	Local clinical audit
National/regional/district	Confidential enquiry into maternal deaths	Confidential enquiry into near misses	National/ regional/ district clinical audit

the facility level and not be possible at the community level. On the other hand, both outcome and process are amenable to review at the facility level. It is unlikely to be possible to review severe complications at the community level because of the complexity of applying a standard and unambiguous definition of 'near miss'. Table 2 summarizes the different possibilities.

These approaches for investigating maternal deaths have been developed mainly for countries where levels of maternal mortality are high. However, the investigation of maternal deaths is also important in settings where maternal mortality is low. Evidence has shown that, even in such settings, many maternal deaths are the result of substandard care and could be prevented.

The importance of 'telling the story'

Most of these approaches are observational studies which take account of the medical and non-medical factors that led to a woman's death. They provide data on individual cases, which, when aggregated together, can show trends or common factors for which remediable action may be possible. They *tell the story* of how individual women died.

Participating in reviews such as those described here, whether by describing one's own contribution to the care of a particular woman, extracting information from the case notes or by assessing the case anonymously, is, in and of itself, a health care intervention. Experience has shown that the use of these approaches can have a major impact on those involved. Often those participating in the review are motivated to change their practice or service delivery, even before the formal publication of the results. These health care workers, who have seen for themselves the benefits from such relatively simple reviews, including the adoption of simple changes in local practice, become advocates for change. They then motivate and enthuse others to undertake similar work and to help spread evidence-based best practice guidance.

Those participating in such reviews also never forget that each woman's death is an individual personal and family tragedy. Neither do they forget she had a unique story to tell. Tracing her path through the community and health care system and describing the actions that might have prevented her death have a meaningful personal effect. In the UK, as long ago as 1954, it was recognized that participating in such a study (in this case a confidential enquiry into maternal deaths) had a 'powerful secondary effect' in that 'each participant in these enquiries, however experienced he or she may be, and whether his or her work is undertaken in a teaching hospital, a local hospital, in the community or the patient's home must have benefited from their educative effect'[12].

Participating in these studies also builds on the natural altruism of individual or teams of health care professionals, who are prepared to freely give their time and effort in order to learn lessons to help save women's lives. These personal experiences lead to self-reflective learning which is as much, or even more a valuable tool for harnessing change as anonymous statistical reporting.

But perhaps one of the most powerful reasons for such reviews, reported by clinicians and midwives in different countries, is the personal and long-lasting impact that the death of a woman known to them has had on their own clinical practice and that of their institution. Most will say that having to seriously evaluate the care given to a particular women, whose face they can still see and whose grieving family they can still remember, changed their clinical practice and subsequently saved many lives.

No name, no blame

A fundamental principle of all the approaches described here is the importance of a confidential, usually anonymous, non-threatening environment in which to describe and analyse the factors leading to individual women's deaths. Ensuring confidentiality leads to an openness in reporting which provides a more complete picture as to the precise sequence of events. Participants, including health care and community workers and family members, should be assured that the sole purpose of the study is to save lives and not to apportion blame. A pre-requisite, therefore, is that strict confidentiality, or anonymity, must be maintained. These reviews seek only to identify failures in the health care system, not to provide the basis for litigation, management sanctions or blame.

Learning lessons is a pre-requisite for action

Learning lessons and acting on the results is the whole purpose of using these approaches. There is no point in committing valuable resources to collecting information that just gathers dust on shelves. The information that is collected must be used to help improve maternal health outcomes and empower health professionals to examine their current practices or those of the facility in which they work. Because action is the ultimate goal of these reviews, it is important that those with the ability to implement the recommended changes actively participate in the process. It therefore needs to be agreed at the outset that the information obtained will be used for action.

The results of these reviews will determine what, if any, avoidable or remediable clinical, health system or community based factors were present in the care provided to the women. The lessons derived will enable health care practitioners and health planners to learn from the errors of the past. They will provide evidence of where the problems are and highlight the areas requiring recommendations for health sector and community action as well as clinical guidelines. The results can form a baseline against which the success of changing practice can be monitored. Therefore, in-built into the system, there should be an objective method to monitor how the recommendations are being implemented. This has two benefits: it provides a stimulus for health sector action; and it reminds the study team to be sure that their recommendations are based on firm evidence.

All of the approaches described here will result in recommendations for change. What is important is that the recommendations made should, particularly in poorer countries, be simple, affordable, effective and widely disseminated. They should also be evidence based. Most of the clinical recommendations likely to emerge will be very similar to the evidence-based guidelines which form part of the WHO's Integrated Management of Pregnancy and Childbirth (IMPAC) tools and these could be adapted for local circumstances and introduced swiftly without the need to start developing guidelines from scratch. (IMPAC is a comprehensive set of norms, standards and tools that can be adapted and applied at the national and district levels in support to country efforts to reduce maternal and perinatal morbidity and mortality. Available from Department of Reproductive Health and Research, WHO, Geneva. Consult the website http://www.who.int/reproductive-health/index.htm for other information.)

To summarize, without the ability to diagnose the problem of why so many of the pregnant women in the world die or suffer severe complications of pregnancy, the opportunity to identify the correct remedial actions for particular women in different circumstances is lost. There is no 'one size fits all solution'. Even though the causes and determinants may be similar, each country, district, facility or community faces a unique set of problems and constraints and requires an individualized approach to overcome these. The philosophy proposed here and the methodologies for audit and case review briefly described are the essential first step in this process. Looking 'Beyond the Numbers' to learn lessons in order to save lives and to reduce the burden of severe maternal and neonatal morbidity is practical, effective and may require little in the way of additional resources. Continually acting on the results of reviews which tell the stories of why mothers died saves the lives of future mothers and babies, and respects and honours those women who died so that some good may come from such a vast number of avoidable tragedies.

The views expressed in this article are those of the author and should not be taken to represent those of the World Health Organization.

References

1   Callaghan W. Epilogue. In Berg C. *et al* (eds) *Strategies to Reduce Pregnancy-Related Deaths: From Identification and Review to Action.* Atlanta, GA: Centres for Disease Control and Prevention, US Department of Health and Human Services, 2001

2   World Health Organization. *Maternal Mortality in 1995. Estimates Developed by WHO, UNICEF and UNFPA.* Geneva: WHO, 2001

3   World Health Organization Regional Office for Africa. *Reducing Maternal Deaths; The Challenge of the New Millennium in the Africa Region.* Congo: World Health Organization Regional Office for Africa, 2002. www.afro.who.int/drh/index.html

4   Ministry of Health Egypt. *National Maternal Mortality Study.* Egypt: Ministry of Health, 1992–1993

5   Why Mothers Die. *The United Kingdom Confidential Enquiries into Maternal Health 1997–99.* London: RCOG Press, 2001

6   Mantel GD, Buchmann E, Rees H, Pattinson RC. Severe acute maternal morbidity: a pilot study of a definition for a near-miss. *Br J Obstet Gynaecol* 1998; **105**: 985–90

7   Waterstone M, Bewley S, Wolfe C. Incidence and predictors of severe obstetric morbidity: case-control study. *BMJ* 2001; **322**: 1089–94

8   World Health Organization. *Beyond the Numbers: Reviewing Maternal Deaths and Complications to Make Pregnancy Safer.* Geneva: WHO, 2004; In press

9   Oxley W, Phillips M, Young J. Maternal mortality in Rochdale. *BMJ* 1935; **304**: 304–7

10 National Institute for Clinical Excellence. *Principles and Practice in Clinical Audit.* London: The National Institute for Clinical Excellence, 2002. http://www.nice.org.uk

11 Website http://www.who.int/reproductive-health

12 The Department of Health. *The Confidential Enquiries into Maternal Deaths in England and Wales 1952–54.* London: Department of Health for England, 1954

Skilled attendants for pregnancy, childbirth and postnatal care

Luc de Bernis, Della R Sherratt, Carla AbouZahr and **Wim Van Lerberghe**

World Health Organization, Geneva, Switzerland

This paper sets out the rationale for ensuring that all pregnant women have access to skilled health care practitioners during pregnancy and childbirth. It describes why increasing access to a skilled attendant, especially at birth, is not only based on legitimate demand and clinical common sense, but is also cost-effective and feasible in resource-poor countries. Skilled attendants need to be supported by a health system providing a legal and policy infrastructure, an effective referral system and the supplies that are necessary for effective care. A skilled attendant providing skilled care will help achieve the goals of reducing both maternal and child mortality. Health care professionals as individual practitioners, leaders and informers have an important role in making this a reality.

Introduction: the case for skilled attendants for pregnancy, birth and the postnatal period

Correspondence to: Della R Sherratt, Midwife, Making Pregnancy Safer, Department of Reproductive Health and Research, World Health Organization, Geneva, Switzerland. E-mail: Sherrattd@who.int

Of all health statistics, those for maternal mortality show the greatest disparity between developing and developed countries: more than 99% of maternal deaths occur in poor countries[1], where women run a lifetime risk of dying from a pregnancy-related complication about 250-fold higher than women in developed countries. Of the 210 million women who become pregnant each year some 30 million, or about 15%, develop complications, which are fatal in 1.7% of cases, giving 529,000 maternal deaths per year. In addition, almost 4 million infants do not survive childbirth or the immediate postnatal period, and millions more are disabled because of inadequately managed pregnancies and births—a situation that has remained almost unchanged for many years[2]. Current studies show that deaths within the first week of life account for almost 40% of all deaths among children under 5 years[3]. Today, we know how to prevent and manage pregnancy-related complications and there is increasing recognition that pregnant women should be assisted by a professional health carer with the necessary skills, drugs, supplies, equipment and back-up, particularly during and immediately following childbirth. In the absence of such professional assistance, women pay a heavy price—maternal ratio rates of 1000–2000 per 100,000 births.

The clinical rationale for skilled care during pregnancy and childbirth is unassailable. Skilled attendants—people with midwifery skills, such as midwives and doctors and nurses who have been trained to proficiency in the skills to manage normal (uncomplicated) pregnancies, childbirth and the immediate postnatal period, and identify, manage or refer complications in the woman and newborn[4]—are best placed to ensure the survival and safety of pregnant women and their infants[5-7]. Whatever their professional title, health professionals functioning as skilled attendants should be able to identify early signs of complications, and offer first-line emergency obstetric care (including emergency newborn care) when needed. Despite the absence of evidence from randomized controlled trials due to the practical and ethical constraints, it is a reasonable working hypothesis that it is better for women and their newborns to have care from a skilled health care worker than from someone without skills. That hypothesis gains strength from the experience of countries that have succeeded in reducing maternal mortality in both the developing and developed world.

Early in the twentieth century, maternal mortality levels in Western Europe and North America were similar to those in the developing countries today. Some countries achieved impressively low maternal mortality very quickly (Sweden, Norway, The Netherlands and Denmark)[8-10]; others were unable to show marked reductions in very high maternal mortality until the Second World War (*e.g.* the USA) or remained between these extremes (*e.g.* England and Wales). The differences between those who managed to lower their maternal mortality rate quickly and those who lagged behind appears to have been in the way in which skilled care was organized. Sweden, Norway, The Netherlands and Denmark focused their efforts on providing skilled care close to where women lived, mainly by strengthening the skills of community midwives. In the USA, on the other hand, a hospital model of care for all births was followed. Maternal mortality remained high despite the fact that women were delivering in health care institutions (usually attended by doctors) because the quality of care was poor and there were high levels of iatrogenic complications, particularly infections[11-13]. More recent examples of countries that have successfully lowered maternal mortality, such as Cuba, Egypt, Iran, Jamaica, Bangladesh (albeit only in Matlab district[14]), Thailand, Sri Lanka and Malaysia[15], demonstrate that maternal mortality can be reduced using a variety of different models of care. Furthermore it is clear that such reductions are possible, even when resources are limited. The common feature in all these countries is that they all focus on ensuring that a skilled attendant attends the majority of births. The Thailand experience in particular shows how providing

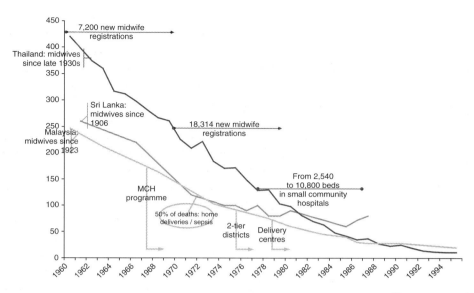

Fig. 1 Maternal mortality since the 1960s in Malaysia, Sri Lanka and Thailand[12] (reproduced with permission).

skilled attendants, in this case midwives, resulted in dramatically reduced maternal and newborn mortality (Fig. 1). In Egypt, higher use of skilled care during delivery was achieved through a dual strategy involving improved quality of care in health facilities coupled with information targeted to decision-making at the household level, which led to an increase in women and families seeking skilled care.

Clinical rationale

There are sound medical reasons why governments should invest in skilled attendants, especially for the time of birth. Most maternal and newborn deaths—with the significant exception of those associated with unsafe abortion which is responsible for an estimated 13% of maternal deaths—occur around the time of childbirth or shortly thereafter (Table 1)[16]. Globally, some 80% of maternal deaths are due to a few direct obstetric

Table 1 Timing of maternal deaths

Time of death	% of all maternal deaths
During pregnancy	24
During delivery	16
After delivery	61

Figures more than 100% due to rounding up to nearest whole numbers.

complications—sepsis, haemorrhage, eclampsia, obstructed labour and unsafe abortion; most could be prevented or managed if the woman had access to a skilled attendant with the necessary back-up and support. The remaining deaths, those caused by underlying conditions exacerbated by pregnancy, *e.g.* severe anaemia, tuberculosis (TB), malaria and HIV/AIDS[17], also require the assistance of a skilled health care provider during pregnancy, birth and the immediate postnatal period for appropriate management and treatment. Complications that result in maternal mortality and morbidity also contribute to the majority of newborn mortality and morbidity. Some of these complications can be prevented with appropriate management of labour and birth (*e.g.* clean birth and monitoring of labour to recognize prolonged and obstructed labour as well as signs of fetal distress). Even when they cannot be prevented, like the vast majority of maternal complications they can be effectively managed. However, this requires health care providers who have the requisite skills, as well as a functional referral system.

Skilled attendants are required to deliver known cost-effective interventions

The World Health Organization (WHO) has identified a number of cost-effective interventions for the management of the major causes of maternal death[18] and has made the information available through the WHO Reproductive Health Library (RHL)[19]. These interventions require a person with midwifery competencies and selective obstetric skills and back-up during the critical period of labour, birth and the immediate post-partum period, in order to prevent, manage or refer in a timely way. The same is true for prevention and management of endemic diseases known to complicate pregnancy, such as malaria, tuberculosis and hepatitis. Managing these conditions requires drugs, equipment and medical skills similar to those needed for the management of obstetric conditions.

Women want skilled assistance at birth

In large parts of the world skilled attendance is not the rule. Table 2 shows currently available data from Demographic and Health Surveys (DHS) on assistance during childbirth by major regional groupings. While the regional aggregations hide important differences both between and within countries, it is clear that doctors attend most births in the Middle East/North Africa and Latin America/Caribbean regions. In sub-Saharan Africa, other categories of professional health care providers (midwives, nurses and other formal health care workers) attended 39% of births, while relatives assisted 27% of births. In Asia, it is the traditional birth attendants (TBAs) who are the largest single group of carers (41% of

Table 2 Attendants at delivery, by region (data from most recent DHS surveys)

Region	Doctor	Other skilled attendant	TBA	Relative	No one	Don't know	Total
Sub-Saharan Africa	5.8	39.1	22.2	26.8	5.9	0.4	100.0
Middle East/North Africa	45.2	21.2	16.2	15.6	1.6	0.3	100.0
Asia	16.6	24.6	40.8	16.4	1.6	0.3	100.0
Latin America/Caribbean	47.8	16.4	24.4	9.7	1.4	0.4	100.0

births), however the regional differences are vast. Sri Lanka, for example, has a very high proportion of births attended by midwives and in Indonesia efforts are currently focused on making midwives available in the rural areas[20] while Thailand, as already mentioned, has made a deliberate and concerted effort to ensure all women have access to maternal care provided by a skilled attendant. Although, in most countries, more and more births benefit from assistance by a health care professional with midwifery skills, sadly, there remain large parts of the world where women have either no one, or only family members, to assist them during childbirth. The situation is worst in sub-Saharan Africa partly due to the devastating effects of HIV/AIDS on the available human resources for all aspects of health care.

Those studying the trends and uses of skilled attendants have noted that the more educated and wealthier women are, the more likely they are to have their births attended by a professional health practitioner[21]. In this regard, it appears women in resource-poor countries are no different from those in rich countries: provided they have the option, they choose the most skilled carers they can find—skilled attendants if these are available, accessible and affordable. Examples abound of women in resource-poor countries who spend much money and effort to go straight to a large referral hospital, even when there is no clinical reason for referral-level care, bypassing the lower levels of care, sometimes even the district hospital, because they expect to get more skilled care.

As Kunst and Houweling graphically represent in their diagram (Fig. 2), in many resource-poor countries as many as 80–90% in the highest economic groups already benefit from a skilled attendant at birth. For the other countries, such options are not yet available, or are no longer an affordable option. Examples from countries such as Tajikistan and Mongolia show what happens when there is rising impoverishment and a breakdown of the health care system—an increasing recourse to home births without skilled attendants—and, in the case of Mongolia between 1991 and 1994, to a rise in maternal mortality ratio from 120 to 210 per 100,000 live births[22]. Unless skilled care is made available at a cost that poor families can afford, many women and their newborns will face

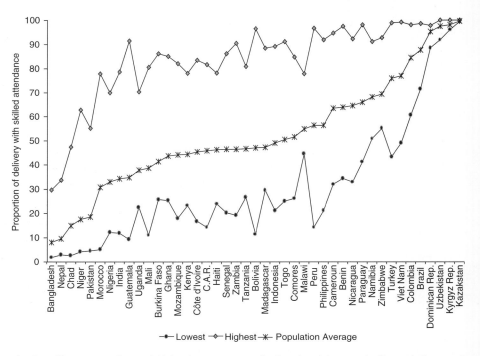

Fig. 2 Delivery attendance (%) in the poorest quintile, the richest quintile and the total population[21] (reproduced with permission).

complications and potential tragedy during the time they need care most, during birth and the period immediately around birth. That this is allowed to continue without outrage, especially from those professionals who purport to have the best interests of women and newborns uppermost, can only be described as tragic.

The limitations of lay referral for obstetric complications

If deaths due to pregnancy-related complications are to be averted, women with all types of complication need to be able to reach appropriate care in a timely manner. Delays in reaching care are often summarized as the 'three delays'—delay in recognizing complications, delay in reaching care and delay in receiving appropriate care at the health facility.

There has been much interest in reducing the first two types of delay for women with complications whose births were attended by lay carers: family members or TBAs, trained or untrained. The term TBA is one around which there is currently a lot of controversy and debate. It is used to define a wide and heterogeneous group of traditional carers most of whom operate in the informal sector, and their individual competencies and skills can vary considerably, as can the names/titles by which they are commonly referred to, depending on the specific country context. Although in some countries it is clear that woman utilize the skills of such carers, research findings indicate that training TBAs is not an effective strategy for reducing maternal mortality. For example, a study comparing maternal mortality and morbidity in two urban populations in Senegal showed that even trained TBAs were unable to accurately recognize signs of complications early, or were unable to make a correct diagnosis and take appropriate action for managing complications[23].

Lay identification of early warning signs is not feasible

Investments in two of the 'three delays', namely early identification of so-called danger-signs or signs of complications and timely self- or community-referral resulted in a focus on strengthening the skills of TBAs, and educating women, families and communities to recognize when to seek medical care. This approach was based on an assumption that early recognition and referral of complications is possible at the household level. This assumes that the woman herself, or family members or TBAs, can acquire the information and knowledge needed for making a timely referral, *i.e.* early detection of complications. Yet, in reality, most pregnancy-related complications, with the exception of bleeding in pregnancy before labour commences, are difficult to recognize until the condition is severe, or are so sudden in onset and quickly progress to become life-threatening that timely referral is difficult to achieve—except for those fortunate enough to have specialized means of transport, or who live close to a referral centre. For example, recognizing early signs and symptoms of severe pre-eclampsia so that appropriate action can be taken is almost impossible without appropriate diagnostic techniques and equipment. Even where complications do start with early signs and symptoms, they are often ignored because they may be considered 'normal'—for example, heavy post-partum bleeding in some cultures is seen as a positive process for purging of impurities in the woman's body[24]. Early recognition of fetal and newborn complications is equally difficult. Thus, reliance on educating women, families and communities to respond to early signs and symptoms, without this being part of a larger strategy for increasing access and utilization of professional skilled care is problematic and may even be morally questionable. Effective timely referral and management of complications requires specific knowledge, skills and training.

Primary health care alone is not sufficient

As with any medical emergency, the chances of survival in the event of an obstetric emergency are directly related to the effectiveness of initial triage—action taken at the time of onset or as close to it as possible. Unfortunately, due to the heavy reliance on primary care since the mid to late 1970s, very little attention has been given in many resource-poor countries to addressing the need to build adequate and appropriate emergency response systems, including referral systems and facilities that can deal with all types of medical emergencies, especially obstetric emergencies[25]. A skilled attendant would however be able to provide appropriate triage and thus help minimize delays in receiving appropriate treatment, as well as institute timely action at all points of the potential delay chain.

Teamwork is crucial

To be effective, the skilled attendant has to work in close collaboration, not only with others in the obstetric team and other health care providers, but also with lay care-givers: TBAs, traditional healers and family members. These lay care-givers play an important social and cultural role, and often control and facilitate access to skilled attendants and referral care[26]. They cannot replace skilled attendants, they do not have the skills or training, nor do they have any mechanisms for regulation and accreditation of their practice. However, where they do function, they should do so as part of the team, operating in close collaboration with, or under the supervision of, a skilled attendant to ensure that women and newborns can access skilled care. In addition, where they exist, traditional healers and TBAs often have local social and cultural knowledge that the skilled attendants can learn from, and so a relation-ship, which is mutually beneficial, is possible and should be developed. For this relationship to work, however, it must be based on mutual trust and respect.

Skilled care is needed during pregnancy as well as at birth

Whilst skilled care during childbirth and management of complications must surely be a priority, safe motherhood and maternal and newborn health programmes should not neglect the potential benefits to be had from some of the elements of antenatal care.

Antenatal care has long been viewed as a screening tool to identify women most at risk of developing severe complications—but recent debates have questioned its efficacy in terms of reducing maternal mortality[27,28]. Despite these limitations as a screening tool, better understanding of fetal growth and development and its relationship to the mother's health has resulted in increased and renewed attention to the benefits of a more 'focused' model of antenatal care, such as the one tested by WHO[29]. For example, tetanus immunization, prevention and treatment of malaria, management of anaemia during pregnancy, and treatment of sexually transmitted infections can significantly improve fetal outcomes (including low birth weight) and maternal health. More recently, the potential of the antenatal period as an entry point for HIV prevention and care, including prevention of mother-to-child transmission of HIV, has led to renewed interest in access to and use of antenatal care services. All this requires care by a skilled professional provider—a skilled attendant.

Besides its direct contribution to better health outcomes, a focused antenatal care model provided by a skilled attendant can also contribute to safer childbirth. First, because women who attend antenatal care are more likely to seek care from a skilled attendant at the time of birth[30,31], particularly if the attendant at the antenatal consultation is the same as the one who also offers care for childbirth. Second, because antenatal care is an opportunity for assisting the woman and her family to make a 'birth and emergency preparedness plan'. Such a plan can help ensure that everyone in the family is familiar with when, why and how to seek immediate medical care as well as the preparations required for and action to be taken when labour commences. Combined with schemes to cover direct and indirect costs of transportation and to ensure that women have access to transport when they need it—irrespective of their ability to pay at the time of need—such 'birth and emergency preparedness plans' can be of great help to women when problems arise[32]. Although any knowledgeable person could assist the family develop these plans, it is crucial for the family to have the opportunity to review the plan with a skilled attendant, and this is considered a fundamental component of the new WHO Antenatal Care Model[33].

Skilled attendants value for money

Skilled care is not only a matter of clinical common sense, but it has advantages in terms of value for money—a critical factor for all countries not just those where economies are flagging or resources are lacking. Cost-savings are not just related to the numbers of deaths averted. Providing women with appropriate skilled care, especially at and around the time of birth, has the potential of reducing the incidence of morbidity. It is estimated that the global burden of disease (measured

Table 3 Cost estimates for using oxytocin for prevention of post-partum haemorrhage in Uganda

		Scenario 1: no preventive intervention	Scenario 2: with preventive intervention
Population	1,094,000		
Pregnancies	64,863		
Incidence of PPH	10%		
Potential cases	6486		
Intervention's effectiveness	50% (3243 fewer cases)		
Unit cost of treatment for PPH		$56	$56
Cost of treatment for cases of PPH		$364,011	$182,006
Savings			$182,006
Total programme cost			$1,800,000
Potential savings[a]			10%

Rounded to nearest whole numbers.

Figures taken from two Districts Iganga and Mbarara.

[a]Actual savings depend on factoring, such as additional costs, savings from all types of complications averted, *etc*.

in terms of disability-adjusted life years[34]) from maternal and newborn complications is approximately 10%. Thus, if cost calculations also included cost-savings to the health sector and health gains to the individual women and their families as a result of averting morbidity as well as mortality, there is little doubt that providing skilled attendants for pregnancy, birth and postnatal care would be shown to be a cost-effective intervention.

Although the evidence remains patchy, the costing studies that are available consistently demonstrate the potential benefit of skilled attendants in terms of costs of treating complications[35]. In Uganda, for example, about 10% of expenditure for maternal health can be avoided through implementing active management of the third stage of labour by a skilled attendant and so avoiding the cost associated with treating such cases[36] (Table 3).

Thus the costs of implementing a skilled attendant strategy can be offset against savings made, especially savings gained from averting complications. In addition, cost can be kept low by implementing quality, low-technology skilled care rather than skilled care in a highly medical referral facility, which should be kept for management of complications.

Finally, the benefits to be gained from implementing a skilled attendant model of care for pregnancy and birth, in terms of strengthening the whole health care system should not be underestimated. A functioning referral system to deal effectively with maternal and newborn complications can be utilized by all others in the community when needed. For example, emergency transportation systems for use by obstetric patients can also be used to transfer non-obstetric emergency cases.

Making it happen—what health professionals can do

Advocacy and action

Health professionals, armed with knowledge and political will, not only can bring this issue to the attention of the appropriate policy-makers, leaders and health planners, but also can advocate for and take positive action at all levels of the health system.

National commitment

By forming alliances with women's groups and with other health professionals, professional associations can bring a unified voice to call for national action to ensure all women and their newborns, including the poorest, have access to a skilled attendant for pregnancy, childbirth and for the postnatal period. The first problem that must be addressed in order to make skilled care available to all is for those in positions of power—especially political leaders—to recognize that reducing maternal and perinatal mortality cannot be addressed only at the primary care level. Lack of minimal life-saving skills and equipment at the first referral level, and inappropriate patient management combined with poor quality of care, can actively contribute to maternal mortality[37].

Improving quality of care

Not only does inadequate and inappropriate care lead to higher incidence of iatrogenic incidents, including leaving women and newborns with severe disability or chronic illness, but it also leads to lack of confidence in the system and low utilization. Although more investment is needed to strengthen the referral facilities within the health system and to ensure that increased access to skilled care goes hand in hand with improved ability of the system to provide quality life-saving care, health providers themselves must become more accountable for the quality of the care they provide. There are many ways in which health professionals can have an important and critical role to play in improving quality of care.

First, it is essential to promote the principles of evidence-based care, including evidence-based decision-making. Health professionals have a duty not only to ensure they themselves keep up-to-date and base their care on sound evidence and clinical reasoning, but should also assist and facilitate others to do the same. Setting clinical protocols and standards based on evidence is essential for any quality improvement initiative.

Secondly, health professionals should try to influence health managers to develop appropriate systems based on evidence, including use of evidence for rational purchasing and use of equipment and drugs. Here WHO has been proactive in making a great deal of the recent evidence for best practice in the field of maternal and newborn health freely available to health practitioners in resource-poor countries—through the various manuals and guidelines, as well as through the provision of Cochrane systematic reviews in the electronic journal *WHO Reproductive Health Library* (RHL). In addition, WHO has been an influential part of the movement which successfully managed to persuade the publishing companies to distribute over 200 medical journals free to resource-poor countries. However, it is the responsibility of each and every professional individual to utilize such evidence and put it into their own practice, as well as promote changes in peers. One example could be to bring the evidence for use of magnesium sulphate as the drug of first choice for control of eclampsia[38], as well as its use in prevention of eclampsia as shown by the result of the recent *MAGPIE* trial, to the attention of those responsible at the national level for the essential medicines list. A recent unpublished review of national essential drug lists by WHO showed that despite the evidence for this low-cost intervention, magnesium sulphate was not on 50% of the national lists reviewed.

One crucial way for health professionals to improve the quality of care is to review regularly and audit their practice. Clinical audit has many positive advantages if the process is undertaken correctly and does not become a blaming or punitive process. Many tools are now available to assist professional practitioners improve their skills. Clinical audit, for example, is one of the several methods discussed in WHO's *Beyond The Numbers*[39]—a guide to help investigate the causes of maternal mortality and near-miss cases in such a way as to lead to improvements of quality of care. WHO South-East Asia Region (WHO SEARO) have produced a set of standards for midwifery practice[40] which also includes a tool for auditing practice, but there are many other tools which can help guide practitioners fulfil this important function and take positive action to improve the quality of care.

Standards are required not just for clinical care

Upgrading of facilities to provide basic or comprehensive obstetric and neonatal care may require both substantial renovation and a programme of regular maintenance. Here again health professionals can both advocate for and be actively involved in developing and implementing evidence-based standards. Standards are required not just for clinical care but also for regular and effective maintenance, cleanliness and management, and for renovating or refurbishment of facilities. Indeed in the latter it is imperative that clinicians are actively involved, as it is at such times when workload activities, patient management systems and even daily routines can be reviewed to improve quality of care and client satisfaction. Too often, clinical staff abdicate the development of such standards to others or they do not foster helpful and collaborative working practices whereby such standards can be developed in a healthy multiprofessional ethos. Unhealthy rivalries can arise between the different health staff and these have an unhelpful and sometimes demoralizing effect on all concerned, as well as leading to poor quality of care.

Team work

All health professionals should be mindful of the importance of working together and that they must operate as team members at two levels, working with other formal health care providers and with the local community, to ensure that all women can access quality maternity services. For services to be truly accessible, all the barriers that impact on utilization must be addressed. Provision of funds for emergency care has been shown to have a positive effect on utilization of services, and although health practitioners cannot be expected to operate such funding schemes, they can advocate and promote such schemes—by helping local leaders and communities explore options for emergency transport systems with local health planners.

Provision of quality maternity care requires a team approach. Whilst the midwife or nurse with midwifery skills can provide care for the woman and her newborn where there are no complications, they must have the support of their medical colleagues—obstetricians or medical doctors with obstetric skills, or at least with surgical skills to be able to undertake a caesarean section. These colleagues must be available at all times in a facility able to manage major complications. Where resources permit, other specialist health providers, social workers, *etc.*, also have an important role to play.

Upgrading skills

To ensure that all women and newborns have access to a skilled attendant at birth there is an urgent need for upgrading the skills of various cadres of health provider based on the available resources and on a 'fitness-for-purpose' curriculum[41]. Strategies to achieve this can include training: (1) nurses in midwifery competencies, (2) general medical staff in basic obstetric surgery, and (3) nurses and midwives in anaesthetic skills. Sometimes it is professional interest groups who, either historically or by accident, erect barriers against others being able to offer appropriate care. Protectionism of professional self-interests can lead to unhelpful conflicts and is counterproductive to removing barriers to providing effective care. The legal and regulatory barriers in particular are often the most difficult to address and can have a negative impact on national action to ensure 'the skilled attendant for all' strategy is implemented. An example of such a barrier with a negative impact is the situations where nurses and midwives are not allowed under national or local regulations to carry out certain life-saving procedures, even when these are taught as part of the pre-service curriculum.

Skilled care for all requires increased coverage

In terms of ensuring there is sufficient, well-qualified and appropriately skilled staff to deliver the services, all health practitioners have an important role in training and supervising less experienced staff, as well as in induction of new staff. It is not only more or better training that is required, although both are crucial, but also more attention is needed to deployment and retention of staff. Individual staff working at the primary level of care cannot be responsible for national policies, but staff working in referral facilities can actively link with their colleagues in the periphery, offering them supportive assistance—inviting them to seminars, updates or in-service activities. In some instances, it may also be possible for staff in referral facilities to share the responsibility of updating staff in the periphery by agreeing to swap positions for a short time, thus allowing peripheral staff the opportunity of spending periods of time working in the referral centres.

Research

Health professionals can also be proactive in research, especially operations research, to explore and critically look at various issues surrounding provision of skilled care—such as mapping where women give birth, whether they have a choice of place of birth and/or type of assistant they have for birth, and which women have access to skilled care, as well as which women are the ones having pregnancy-related complications. All of these and much more need careful investigation to be able to understand some of the complex contextual issues impinging on access to, and utilization of, skilled care. For example, there may be a number of advantages in suggesting that all women give birth in a health care facility, especially where there is a shortage of skilled attendants. However, this proposal needs careful consideration, not only on the grounds of denying women the right to choose, but also on feasibility. The cost of building and maintaining large maternity facilities, and the potential that exists for facility care leading to over-medicalization of care also need to be addressed.

Challenges for health professionals and their associations

It should not be underestimated that health practitioners in resource-poor countries face numerous and difficult barriers to providing effective evidence-based skilled care in pregnancy, childbirth and the postnatal period. Faced with declining national economies and lacking a good standard of remuneration, many health practitioners will be tempted to seek employment in the private sector, or even to leave the health service to take up other work that offers them better economic rewards. This situation will only be exacerbated where poor working relationships exist and where there is not a sense of shared understanding and pooling of resources, including pooling of political will and action to begin to address the situation.

Whilst individuals may be helpless to impact on the development of 'staff-friendly' human policies, professional associations can however work together to advocate for, and assist in, the development of equitable human resources policies at all levels. In addition, those professions with greater political voice can collaborate with those with less power and voice, so that the service as a whole can be improved to benefit all women and newborns.

Women's empowerment

In many countries, the greatest barrier to creating an enabling environment where 'skilled care for all' can become a reality is the low status of women and their lack of opportunities to begin to demand skilled care and hold governments accountable for the services they receive. Here again, health professionals can contribute to changing the general lack of women's political power and opportunities to have their concerns heard at all levels of decision-making, by bringing to the attention of all the need for better education of girls and women and the contribution this makes to maternal and newborn health[42]. Skilled attendants–health professionals, at both the individual provider–client interaction level, but also at a collective level, have an important opportunity to begin to influence and promote an empowering climate for women.

At the provider–client level practitioners can give more attention to providing support and education to women and can encourage women to make informed decisions about their care. This will require practitioners to adopt a partnership model of care—one where women and their families are seen as legitimate decision-makers in their health care.

At the collective level, health professionals can act as women's advocates by working with, supporting, or even encouraging the setting-up of local women's networks, postnatal support groups, *etc.*, to lobby for skilled care and improvements to maternity services. In addition, health professionals can assist women by ensuring that the issues that hinder access to skilled care for all are brought to the attention of the general public and political leaders, with a demand for political action to help reduce maternal and newborn mortality and morbidity. In particular, the needs of the poorest must be addressed, as it is they who are too frequently too busy and burdened with the daily concerns of living to be able to politically advocate for their own needs. They are also among the voiceless and are frequently uninformed about the need for skilled care and about how to access such care even when it does exist.

To meet the human resource demands to ensure that there are sufficient skilled attendants to be able to offer all women and their newborns access to skilled care requires a more systematic approach than has hitherto been the norm. Professionals, professional groups (such as midwives, nurse-midwives, nurses and obstetricians) and their associations can assist by:

- Working together—not simply protecting their own territory.

- Developing and instigating clear codes of conduct, with professional accountability for provision of quality care.

- Advocate for the removal of barriers that place women and newborns at risk because of inadequate levels of care, including lack of coverage by a skilled attendant.

- Advocate for adequate and appropriate recompense for skilled attendants working in rural areas (including the need for career enhancement opportunities), as well as attention to be given to security and protection issues, especially for the lone female workers.

Finally, professionals and their associations have the greatest potential for making an impact on *quality of care*, especially by making sure that care provision conforms to national and international standards. The challenge they face is also to ensure that care is acceptable to the local population. Given the competing demands for resources at the household level, it will not be possible to increase demand for, and thus access to and utilization of, skilled care without addressing costs to the individual. Greater attention therefore needs to be given to educating communities that investments for strengthening the emergency referral system will not only benefit women and newborns, but that such systems can also be utilized for dealing with other medical emergencies, accidents, *etc.* This will only be possible, however, if the community members can see for themselves that the care they are offered does lead to noticeable results, including the feeling that they are treated with dignity and respect when accessing services.

Above all, to implement a skilled attendant model of care for pregnancy, childbirth and the postnatal period, health practitioners must engage with local communities—first to identify what are the local customs, beliefs and behaviours surrounding pregnancy, childbirth and postnatal including early newborn care, and then to address these with local leaders, community influencers, *etc*. In many instances, local beliefs and customs that are not harmful can be incorporated sympathetically in modern western practices; these issues are dealt with in greater detail in the paper by Portela and Santarelli in this volume. Health professionals must recognize that women's desire for safe, yet respectful and friendly care—care that takes account of their emotional, cultural and spiritual needs—is possible, but to do so takes ingenuity and a willingness on the side of the health professional to be flexible.

Conclusion

Global health policy has long overlooked the need to develop effective systems for dealing with medical emergencies, including obstetric emergencies. This has contributed to the lack of successfully reducing maternal mortality. Evidence shows that improving the education and training of health care workers with midwifery skills is an important first step in any maternal mortality reduction strategy, and can begin even before other improvements to the health care system have been achieved—but both are needed. Sadly, previous strategies have not paid attention to either building a midwifery cadre or building good health systems, in particular, systems that can adequately deal with obstetric emergencies. If the millennium goals of improving health of women, for which reduction in maternal mortality is paramount, and for reducing child mortality, for which greater attention is required through reducing newborn deaths, then concerted action is urgently needed to promote and achieve increased access to, and utilization of, skilled care for pregnancy, especially for childbirth and the immediate postnatal period. Skilled care requires a health professional with midwifery skills who is equipped with the essential drugs and is equipped and supported by a policy and regulatory framework to allow them to function effectively. At the very least, all skilled attendants must be able to recognize early signs of complications, provide first-line obstetric management (including first-line management of newborn complications) and make an effective timely referral to a facility where the complication can be appropriately managed.

It is clear that all the above is not easy to achieve, but the consequences of not achieving them should be kept in mind—the unacceptable number of women, newborns and families who will continue to be subject to such human tragedy, the costs of which are almost incalculable, the suffering of those left almost inconsolable and, most tragic of all, the fact that much of this suffering could have been averted. Thus, providing a skilled attendant for all women and their newborns in pregnancy and childbirth needs to be seen by all as a priority at national and global levels, especially by those concerned with human life, health and the rights of all individuals to live a healthy, sexual and reproductive life, *i.e.* health practitioners working in the field of reproductive health care.

The views expressed in this article are those of the author and should not be taken to represent those of the World Health Organization.

References

1   World Health Organization. *Maternal Mortality in 1995: Estimates Developed by WHO, UNICEF, UNFPA.* Geneva: WHO, 2000

2   World Health Organization. *Research on Reproductive Health at WHO: Biennial Report 2000–2001.* Geneva: WHO, 2002

3   Tinker A, Ranson E. *Healthy Mothers and Healthy Newborns. The Vital Link: Policy Perspectives on Newborn Health.* Saving Newborn Lives and Policy Reference Bureau, 2002

4   WHO/ICM/FIGO. *Skilled Attendants—The Way Forward.* Geneva: WHO (forthcoming)

5   Hogberg U, Wall S, Brostrom G. The impact of early medical technology of maternal mortality in late XIXth century Sweden. *Int J Gynecol Obstet* 1986; **24**: 251–61

6   World Health Organization. *Joint WHO/UNICEF Statement on Maternal Care for the Reduction of Perinatal and Neonatal Mortality.* Geneva: WHO, 1986

7   World Health Organization. *Mother–Baby Package: A Practical Guide to Implementing Safe Motherhood in Countries.* Document WHO/FHE/MSM/94.11. Maternal Health and Safe Motherhood Programme, Division of Family Health, 1994

8   Loudon I. *Death in Childbirth. An International Study of Maternal Care and Maternal Mortality 1800–1950.* London: Oxford University Press, 1992

9   Loudon I. Maternal mortality in the past and its relevance to the developing world today. *Am J Clin Nutr* 2000; **72**: 241S–246S

10   Loudon I. Midwives and the quality of maternal care. In: Marland H, Rafferty AM (eds) *Midwives, Society and Childbirth: Debates and Controversy of the Modern Period.* London and New York: Routledge, 1997; 180–200

11   De Bouwere V, Tonglet R, Van Lerberghe W. Strategies for reducing maternal mortality in developing countries: what can we learn from the history of the industrialised West? *Trop Med Int Health* 3: 771–82

12   Van Lerberghe W, De Brouwere V. Of blind alleys and things that have worked: history's lessons on reducing maternal mortality. In: De Brouwere V, Van Lerberghe W (eds) *Safe Motherhood Strategies: A Review of the Evidence. Stud Health Serv Organ Policy* 2001; **17**: 7–33

13   Porges RF. The response of the New-York Obstetrical Society to the report by the New-York Academy of Medicine on maternal mortality, 1933–34. *Am J Obstet Gynecol* 1985; **152**: 642–9

14   Ronsmans C *et al.* Decline in maternal mortality in Matlab, Bangladesh: a cautionary tale. *Lancet* 1997; **350**: 1810–4

15   Pathmanathan I *et al. Investing Effectively in Maternal and Newborn Health in Malaysia and Sri Lanka.* Washington, DC, USA: World Bank, 2003

16   Koblinski M *et al. Issues in Programming for Safe Motherhood.* Arlington, VA: MotherCare, 2000

17 Pradhan EK *et al*. Risk of death following pregnancy in rural Nepal. *Bull WHO* 2002; **80**: 887–91

18 World Health Organization. *Global Action for Skilled Attendants for Pregnant Women*. Appendix 2. Geneva: WHO, 2002.

19 World Health Organization. *WHO Reproductive Health Library No 6*. Geneva: Department of Reproductive Health and Research, WHO, 2003

20 Ronsmans C *et al*. Evaluation of a comprehensive home-based midwifery programme in South Kalimantan, Indonesia. *Trop Med Int Health* 2001; **6**: 799–810

21 Kunst A, Houweling T. A global picture of poor–rich differences in the utilisation of delivery care. In: De Brouwere V, Van Lerberghe W (eds) *Safe Motherhood Strategies: A Review of the Evidence*. *Stud Health Serv Organ Policy* 2001; **17**: 297–315

22 World Bank. *Mongolia: Poverty Assessment in a Transition Economy*. Report EA2RS. Washington, DC: World Bank, 1996

23 De Bernis L *et al*. Maternal morbidity and mortality in two different populations in Senegal: a prospective study (MOMA survey). *Br J Obstet Gynaecol* 2000; **107**: 68–74

24 Okolocha C *et al*. Socio-cultural factors in maternal morbidity and mortality: a study in semi-urban community in southern Nigeria. *J Epidemiol Commun Health* 1998; **52**: 293–7

25 Razzak J, Kellermann A. Emergency care in developing countries: is it worthwhile? *Bull WHO* 2002; **80**: 900–4

26 World Health Organization. TBAs—an important link in the chain. In: *Safe Motherhood: A Newsletter of Worldwide Activity* 2002; **29**: 5

27 Villar J, Bergsjø P. Scientific basis for the content of routine antenatal care. I. Philosophy, recent studies and power to eliminate or alleviate adverse maternal outcomes. *Acta Obstet Gynecol Scand* 1997; **76**: 1–14

28 Bergsjø P. What is the evidence for the role of antenatal care strategies in the reduction of maternal mortality and morbidity? In: De Brouwere V, Van Lerberghe W (eds) *Safe Motherhood Strategies: A Review of the Evidence*. *Stud Health Serv Organ Policy* 2001; **17**: 35–54

29 Carroli G *et al*. (for the WHO Antenatal Care Trial Research Group). WHO systematic review of randomised controlled trials of routine antenatal care. *Lancet* 2001; **357**: 1565–70

30 Bloom S *et al*. Does antenatal care make a difference to safe delivery? A study in urban Uttar Pradesh, India. *Health Policy Plann* 1999; **14**: 28–48

31 Caldwell J, Reddy P, Caldwell P. The social component of mortality decline: an investigation in Southern India employing alternative methodologies. *Popul Stud* 1983; **37**: 185–201

32 Moore M. *Safer Motherhood 2000: Toward a Framework for Behaviour Change to Reduce Maternal Deaths*. The Communication Initiative, 2000, available at: http://www.comminit.com/misc/safer_motherhood.html; last accessed October 2002

33 World Health Organization. *Antenatal Care Randomized Trail: Manual for Implementation of the New Model*. Geneva: WHO, 2002

34 World Health Organization. *The World Health Report 2002: Reducing Risks, Promoting Health Life*. Geneva: WHO, 2002

35 Borghi J. What is the cost of maternal health care and how can it be financed? In: De Brouwere V, Van Lerberghe W (eds) *Safe Motherhood Strategies: A Review of the Evidence*. *Stud Health Serv Organ Policy* 2001; **17**: 247–96

36 Weissman E *et al*. *Uganda Safe Motherhood Programme Costing Study*. Document WHO/RHR/99.9. Geneva: Department of Reproductive Health and Research, WHO, 1999

37 Sundari TK. The untold story: How health care systems in developing countries contribute to maternal mortality. *Int J Health Serv* 1992; **22**: 513–28

38 Eclampsia Trial Collaborative Group. Which anticonvulsant for women with eclampsia? Evidence from the collaborative eclampsia trial. *Lancet* 1995; **345**: 1455–63

39 World Health Organization. *Beyond the Numbers: Reviewing Maternal Deaths and Complications to Make Pregnancy Safer*. Geneva: WHO; In press

40 World Health Organization. *Standards of Midwifery Practice for Safe Motherhood*. New Delhi: WHO SEARO, 2000

41 Sherratt DR. Why women need midwives for safe motherhood. In: Berer M, Sundari Ravindran TK (eds) *Safe Motherhood Initiatives: Critical Issues*. *Reprod Health Matters* 2000; 227–38

42 Elo I. Utilization of maternal health care services in Peru: the role of women's education. *Health Transit Rev* 1992; **2**: 49–61

Empowerment of women, men, families and communities: true partners for improving maternal and newborn health

A Portela* and **C Santarelli†**

*The Making Pregnancy Safer Initiative, Department of Reproductive Health and Research, World Health Organization, Geneva, Switzerland and †Enfants du Monde, Geneva, Switzerland

Based on the Health Promotion approach, the Making Pregnancy Safer initiative has proposed a strategic framework for working with individuals, families and communities to improve maternal and newborn health. The aims are to contribute to the empowerment of women, families and communities to increase their influence and control over maternal and newborn health, as well as to increase access to and utilization of quality skilled care. The framework has identified those strategies and interventions that target the factors known to contribute to health inequalities and poor maternal and newborn health. While empowerment is an aim of the framework, it is also considered a means. Emphasis is placed on the processes and the quality of the processes rather than just on the actions themselves. The authors in this paper would like to contribute to ongoing discussions about the 'how' of working with women, men, families and communities for improved maternal and newborn health.

Background

Correspondence to:
A Portela, Making Pregnancy Safer initiative (MPR), Department of Reproductive Health and Research (RHR), World Health Organization, 20 Avenue Appia, CH-1211 Geneva 27, Switzerland. E-mail: portelaa@who.int

Experience over the past decade has shown that no single intervention is by itself sufficient to improve maternal and newborn health and reduce morbidity and mortality. What is needed is a continuum of care throughout pregnancy, childbirth and the postnatal period[1]. To be effective, the continuum should extend from care in the household, to care provided by the skilled attendant[a] at the primary care level, including the first-level facility, to care provided at the referral facility. The development of this continuum requires commitment, cooperation and interaction between the different levels of care and between the different care providers. Efforts should focus on building capacities at the individual, family and community level to assure appropriate self-care, prevention and care-seeking behaviour. Concurrently, efforts should focus on building the capacity of health care delivery to define and adapt the needed interventions and services and assure that they are

British Medical Bulletin, Vol. 67 © The British Council 2003; all rights reserved

available, acceptable and of high quality, particularly for the poor and most vulnerable. Political commitment and inter-sectoral collaboration form part of the context for the effective development of the continuum.

A framework for working with individuals, families and communities

The WHO Making Pregnancy Safer initiative was launched in 2000 to enhance WHO's efforts in Safe Motherhood. The initiative is oriented to assist countries in strengthening their health systems, to develop evidence-based interventions that target the major causes of maternal and newborn mortality and morbidity, with a focus on reaching the poor. Working with individuals, families and communities is considered a critical link in strengthening the recommended continuum of care. Equally, it is recognized that the availability of quality services alone will not produce the desired health outcomes when there is no possibility to be healthy, to make healthy lifestyle decisions and moreover, to be able to act on those decisions. Health gains as well as healthy lives require more than the provision of services. Individual and collective capacities, as well as other determinants of health, cannot be ignored.

Based on the Health Promotion approach as outlined in the Ottawa Charter[2], the Making Pregnancy Safer initiative has proposed a strategic framework for working with individuals, families and communities to improve maternal and newborn health[3]. The aims are to contribute to the empowerment of women, families and communities[b] to increase their influence and control of maternal and newborn health, as well as to increase access and utilization of quality skilled care[c] by women and their families. The framework (Fig. 1) has identified those strategies and interventions that target the factors known to contribute to health inequalities and poor maternal and newborn health.

Priority interventions

A set of promising interventions (Table 1) to achieve the aims mentioned above, identified both in the literature and from experience, have been organized into four priority areas:

1   Developing capacities of women, families and communities to stay healthy, make healthy decisions and respond to obstetric and neonatal emergencies

2   Increasing awareness of women, families and communities of their sexual and reproductive rights, and of the needs and potential problems related to maternal and newborn health

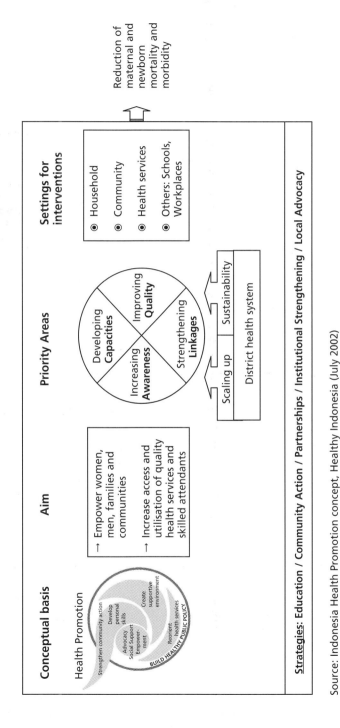

Source: Indonesia Health Promotion concept, Healthy Indonesia (July 2002)

Fig. 1 Strategic framework for the development of individual, family and community (IFC) interventions.

Table 1 Overview of interventions in the priority areas

Priority areas of intervention	Developing **CAPACITIES** to stay healthy, make healthy decisions and respond to obstetric and neonatal emergencies	Increasing **AWARENESS** of the rights, needs and potential problems related to maternal and newborn health	Strengthening **LINKAGES** for social support between women, families and communities and with the health delivery system	Improving **QUALITY** of care, health services and interactions with women and communities
Intervention topics	Self-care	Human rights	Community financial and transport schemes	Community involvement in quality care
	Care-seeking behaviour	The role of men and other influentials	Maternity waiting homes	Social support during childbirth
	Birth and emergency preparedness	Community epidemiological surveillance and maternal-perinatal death audits	Roles of traditional birth attendants within the health system	Interpersonal and intercultural competence of health care providers

3 Strengthening linkages for social support between women, men, families and communities and with the health care delivery system

4 Improving quality of care, health services and health provider interactions with women, men, families and communities

Local context and resources will ultimately decide the interventions to be implemented. Initial assessments will assist in determining priorities. However, a comprehensive strategy, with interventions from each one of the four priority areas, is recommended. Increased capacities and awareness of women, families and communities need to be developed while strengthening linkages in the communities and between the communities and health services. Also, the development of interventions at the household and community level will not achieve its full effect if maternal and newborn health services are not available or responsive to the culture and needs. In sum, an integrated approach is needed that maximizes the benefits of a range of activities, planned and implemented internally within the health sector with other sexual and reproductive health programmes, and externally with other sectors.

Empowerment approaches

While empowerment is an aim of the framework, it is also considered a means, developed at two levels that interact and affect each other[4]:

1 At an individual level, efforts are aimed at increasing resources like knowledge, cognitive capacities, health competencies and the capacity and confidence to make healthy lifestyle choices

2 At a collective or community level, efforts are aimed at applying skills and resources collectively to meet the collective needs, including structural changes to the environment to improve access to social, economic and political resources

In sum, empowerment is an ongoing process of enabling individuals and groups to improve capacities, to critically analyse situations and to take actions to improve those situations[5].

The emphasis is placed on the processes and the quality of the processes rather than just on the actions themselves. Thus, as we look to strengthen the body of information and evidence related to the strategies and priority interventions in the proposed framework, we are also looking to improve understanding of the underlying processes that lead to the desired outcomes.

The authors of this study would like to contribute to ongoing discussions about the 'how' of working with women, men, families and communities for improved maternal and newborn health. Examples of interventions and strategies from the above-mentioned framework are presented applying an empowerment approach (with a focus on pregnancy as an intervention period). Each of the scenarios is grounded in a vision of the health care delivery system and health care providers entering into a reciprocal relationship with women, families and communities where the exchange of information, identification of problems and development of solutions is an ongoing process. Thus, the discussion will ultimately lead us to a reflection on roles and responsibilities. Many will also argue, and rightly so, that in this reflection, empowerment of health care providers must also be considered.

Shared decision-making for maternal and newborn health

The principles of informed decision-making are not new in the field of sexual and reproductive health. These principles have been fundamental tenets of quality family planning services for decades[6]. One of the stated criteria of Women-Friendly Health Services[7] focuses on empowerment of users and respect for their rights, including the right to choice. Yet, it is difficult to find an emphasis on decision-making or problem-solving processes or direct references to this terminology within evaluations of maternal and newborn health programmes in lower-resource settings. Furthermore, although informed decision-making has been embraced as a central focus of modern maternity care in Western and developed countries, evaluations have shown that this has not necessarily been translated into practice[8].

Frequently, maternal and newborn health programmes include components to develop health care providers' inter-personal communication skills. Yet, many programmes in implementation continue to put emphasis on the modality of information giving. The word 'counselling'—which is to provide support for decision-making and problem-solving—is often used interchangeably with providing advice and recommendations. An emphasis is currently given to a good client–provider interaction, highlighting the importance of a dynamic two-way interaction and the woman's active participation[9]. However, a truly empowering encounter would assure that the woman (and her family) would not only receive appropriate information and interact with the health service provider. She would also have the opportunity to analyse the information in relation to her individual situation and life experiences, plan what to do next and explore solutions to the different health issues[d,10–12].

The principle of informed decision-making could be usefully applied in an intervention to increase birth and emergency preparedness[e], identified as a key component of antenatal care[13]. The key elements of a plan to prepare for birth or the eventuality of an obstetric complication (see Table 2) require that, at a minimum, the health care provider works with the pregnant woman to explore the different possibilities, so she can begin to identify the most feasible solutions. For example, the health provider may consider that it is best that the woman give birth in a facility, based on her health status or on an identified obstetric condition. One way for this to become a reality is if the woman was supported in thinking out all of the related issues pertinent to her and her family: does she prefer the care in the recommended facility, how could she get there, who would take care of her home and children, what are the related expenses, how could they meet these expenses, *etc.*

Table 2 Some key elements of a birth and emergency (obstetric and neonatal) plan

- Selecting a birth location (home, health centre or hospital)

- Identifying the location of the closest appropriate care facility, in case of emergency

- Identifying a skilled attendant

- Identifying a companion for the delivery and for emergency

- Identifying support for care of the home and children during delivery and emergency

- Planning for funds for birth-related and emergency expenses

- Arranging transport for facility-based birth and in case of emergency

- Having adequate supplies for the delivery (depending if at home, in a health centre or hospital): a clean delivery kit, clean cloths, clean water (and a way to heat that water), clothes for mother and baby, soap, food and water for the mother and the companion

- Identifying a compatible blood donor in case of haemorrhage

Adapted from: WHO[14] and Moore[13].

Further, given household decision-making processes, the woman more than likely will need support to discuss the plan with her partner and/or other key decision-makers in the household[f]. This may imply inviting the partner or a family member to the next antenatal care session, or having a card that outlines the issues to be resolved. A feasible final plan could only be developed after this interaction at the household level. Providing support to plan for birth and to be prepared for emergencies may not always lead to the recommendation initially envisioned by the health provider. However, birth and emergency preparedness efforts can lead to a decrease in the delays in decision-making for reaching care when needed and an increase in the use of services. And as an empowerment process, based on informed decision-making, the process will also provide the woman and her family with additional capacities to influence and improve health.

A question may arise as to the viability of implementing informed decision-making principles in the busy antenatal care setting. Lack of time is often cited as an impediment. But the time dedicated to an effective antenatal intervention may in the long run decrease time required at another moment in the progression of the chain of maternal care. Research[9,15,16] (extracted from areas other than maternal and newborn health, such as family planning, general practice, hormone replacement therapy, cancer treatment, *etc.*) shows that the time invested in this type of approach could in fact lead to greater satisfaction of the woman with the quality of services, increased understanding of the health situation and increased compliance/continuance/adherence[g]. Increased research is needed to study the details of the applications of this approach within maternal and newborn health, and specifically for birth and emergency preparedness, as well as measurement of the desired outcomes of empowerment and increased use of skilled care.

Another question that may arise relates to the development of health provider skills to engage in an informed decision-making process. We also need to consider health care providers' attitudes and beliefs related to entering into this type of encounter with the woman and her family. Pilot studies and research continue for the development of models to support the development of health care providers' skills and attitudes[10,11,17–19]. Research and other experiences are also being developed looking at the processes and skills of the woman or the client in empowering interactions[19,20]. Efforts should be made to gather and systematize this information, and assure its widespread distribution for increased discussion and application of the lessons learned.

Ultimately, birth and emergency preparedness as an intervention must be considered within a package of interventions[h]. In order to involve other decision-makers in the community and reach women who do not receive antenatal care, some programmes have developed birth preparedness for health workers at the community level[i]. A complementary process of dialogue and building partnership with the community, based on the principles of a reciprocal relationship, may be useful in certain contexts in order to discuss maternal and newborn health needs and the importance of skilled care for births and obstetric complications, postnatal care of the mother and newborn and neonatal complications[21]. The community can also be approached to discuss solutions to obstacles to seeking this needed care, including identification of danger signs, transport schemes, financing schemes, *etc.*

Finally, many of the other recommendations provided to women in antenatal care (postnatal care and care of the newborn as well) could also benefit from the application of the principles of informed decision-making, which despite the result, respects her final choice. This would include those recommendations related to self-care in the household, including increased nutrition, reduced workload activities, iron supplementation compliance and others. All will also require efforts to increase family and community support, but the main concern should be to make sure that programmes advance with the central objective of supporting the woman to take better care of herself and her baby.

Health education approaches

Most community health programmes, as well as the education and communication approaches applied, focus on convincing specified groups to adopt a desired behaviour[5,22]. Many of these models are based on behavioural and social cognitive theories and on a premise that development problems, including poor health, are primarily rooted in a lack of knowledge[23].

Thus, efforts have concentrated on increasing knowledge and changing behaviour for the recommended practices for maternal and newborn health. During pregnancy alone, there are a range of desired behaviours ranging from self-care in the household to preventive measures to care-seeking behaviour for childbirth and emergencies. Yet different evaluations of these efforts often show an increase in knowledge, without the corresponding changes in practice. One possible explanation for this gap is that the input is not sufficiently related to the existing knowledge of people. As a result, neither true appropriation of knowledge nor long-term behaviour change nor local ownership of the processes occurs. Thus, it is inherent that these approaches do not lead to empowerment.

Therefore, a different approach to health education is proposed for discussion to reduce the knowledge–behaviour gap and for empowerment to occur. In this approach, priority is placed on appropriation of knowledge and development of cognitive capacities, rather than a simple increase in knowledge. The approach is based on socio-interactionist theory, which has become the theoretical and experimental basis of current approaches used in formal education, with children and adults, in settings of higher and lower resourced countries.

The socio-interactionist theory emphasizes that the central element in intellectual and psychological development and the learning process is the 'zone of proximal development'. This zone is defined as the distance between the level of current development and the more advanced level of potential development that comes into existence in interactions between more and less capable participants[24]. A key principle for the design of health education processes lies in the effective use of the zone of proximal development, and the identification of existing knowledge and capacities. It recognizes that cognitive development is more efficient in a situation of social interaction.

Another key element of the theory relates to the fact that knowledge, thoughts and the associated practices are socially, historically, institutionally and culturally situated, defined and shared. Thus, external inputs or new knowledge, introduced as untied and unarticulated pieces whose production and coherence are situated outside of the group or community receiving them, cannot be effectively integrated. Individuals receiving this external knowledge do not have the social, linguistic and cultural background to interpret and correctly decode this input.

Also when presenting new knowledge, the strong relationship between thought and language should be taken into account. Socio-interactionist research has demonstrated that one provides resource to the other; language being essential in forming thoughts and in determining personality features[25].

In health education processes, we often simply translate information or 'messages' into the local or popular language, without considering that the structure of language itself and concepts are particular to each society and culture[26]. More attention must be given to this and to finding common words to truly assure that the new concepts are understandable. When a direct translation may not be possible, common words must be identified to form the conceptual basis. A glossary should be created to form a true understanding.

A process of critical debate must occur where existing knowledge confronts new knowledge[j]. New knowledge must be examined according to its pertinence in relation to the socio-cultural context. Phases of deconstruction, decontextualization and subsequent construction and contextualization must occur in the process[27,28]. What is proposed is in fact not the introduction of knowledge but the creation of knowledge (see Table 3).

By understanding and using the socio-interactionist approach, the learning process can be more efficient than with those methodologies that focus on providing information, repetition of messages or imitation of behaviours. This approach also permits the development of superior

Table 3 Key principles of a socio-interactionist approach

- The educational process should start from the participants' knowledge (texts and representations) in order to strengthen or weaken it, present and analyse new external knowledge and create a new knowledge derived from the confrontation of both sets of knowledge.

- The educational process should enable a conceptual attainment of knowledge as well as abilities to further acquire knowledge, in order to permit an autonomous intellectual capacity to continue one's own education. This can be summarized as learning to learn.

- Knowledge expressed and learned has to be linked to social, historical and cultural realities.

- The educational process should be a learning experience that allows the participant to be responsible for his/her own development, in order to reinforce the capacity for critical analysis of his/her own formation and the formation of the other participants.

capacities such as autonomy, critical reflection, social values, establishing a dialectical dynamic between psychological capacities, language and socio-historic-cultural influences.

It is in fact central to the socio-interactionist approach that the learning process allows for not only the development of knowledge but also the development of cognitive capacities used in the integration, the search and the construction of new knowledge, useful for the current process and for future learning processes. By doing so, the approach can contribute to empowerment.

Different approaches and models have been developed based on principles of socio-interactionism. For example, the 'Pedagogy of the Text' (PdT)[k] is an educational approach based on these principles, including the most up-to-date knowledge and relevant research from a number of sciences, including linguistics (textual linguistics), psychology (social inter-activity), pedagogy and didactics. PdT is currently being applied and tested in several countries of Latin America, the Middle East and Africa[l]. The Swiss NGO Enfants du Monde has begun discussing the application of the PdT in maternal and newborn health programmes with national authorities and local and international NGOs in Haiti and Guatemala.

There are different moments in health education components of maternal and newborn health programmes when such an approach can be applied. Some examples include: (a) information and 'message' development—an approach to create knowledge which is socially and culturally situated could serve as a basis for the development of information to be included in educational materials, mass media campaigns and training materials; (b) raising community awareness—the approach can serve as a basis for discussions with communities on maternal and newborn health problems and developing solutions; (c) training of health care providers—such an approach can also be used for the development of curricula content and the learning process for developing their knowledge, capacities and skills.

Other experiences exist which apply concepts similar to those outlined above; some examples include participatory research, community-driven quality approaches and community-action cycles[29]. Community dialogue (between the community and the health programme) is an innovative methodology that can serve to improve mutual understanding and increase awareness of the reality, perspective and conditions of the other party. It recognizes the importance of current knowledge as a starting point, of introducing information on maternal and newborn health needs for discussion and debate, and of the central role of communities in decisions and actions that influence their health and well-being[30–33]. Bolivia has developed different experiences utilizing approaches based on community dialogue, participation and problem-solving. Programmes would benefit from learning more about these experiences, both through a more rigorous evaluation of the methodologies and outcomes and through documentation and discussion of the processes developed.

Future directions

There are several implications of embracing the approaches and principles outlined above that challenge how health programmes generally work with communities. First is to consider how to develop an open attitude in health programmes and service providers, as stated earlier in this document, to accepting a reciprocal relationship with women, families and communities where the exchange of information, identification of problems and development of solutions is an ongoing process. An empowerment approach questions the approaches which most health care providers are trained to apply. New knowledge and information needs to be presented for discussion and debate with women and communities. Decision-making/problem-solving must be a shared responsibility. These are proposed if appropriation of knowledge and the development of capacities are to occur. For some health care professionals, it may be difficult to appreciate the expertise and abilities brought by women and communities into this reciprocal relationship. Different skills, time pressures, existing attitudes, lack of motivation, programme structures and a biomedical culture which dictates a more authoritative relation with 'clients' are some of the factors that can limit broader application of empowering approaches.

Second, these approaches also imply a new role for health care providers and programmes that engage in health education and interaction with the community. The emphasis within an empowerment approach would now lie on facilitation and dialogue and creating knowledge rather than providing the messages and the solutions. Thus, programmes may seek to build health professionals' capacities in these areas as well as strengthen partnerships with other agencies and sectors with more experience in applying these skills.

Finally, there is a need for increased research to study the applications of empowerment approaches within maternal and newborn health programmes. As mentioned above, research should support a better understanding of the processes as well as the outcomes of such interventions (with individuals, families and communities) on knowledge, practices, use of skilled care and empowerment at the individual and collective levels. An evidence-based approach is called upon for effective policy and programming for safe motherhood[34]. This would apply to all levels of the continuum of care. At the individual, family and community level, there are lessons learned about what does not work or what limits programmes from achieving their full potential. Let us now work to build the evidence based on the promising interventions and strategies for building the longer-term capacities.

Bringing together women, families and communities with health care providers is not an easy process. However, sufficient evidence exists to demonstrate that, unless they begin to work more closely together, the goals for maternal and newborn health, including the reduction in morbidity and mortality, cannot be achieved.

The views expressed in this article are those of the authors and should not be taken to represent those of the World Health Organization or Enfants du Monde.

Acknowledgements

The authors would like to extend their appreciation to those who have contributed to the development of this discussion, particularly Antonio Faundez, Gwyneth Lewis, Mona Moore, Edivanda Mugrabi, Della Sherratt and Paul Van Look.

Notes

a   Skilled attendants are 'people with midwifery skills, such as midwives and doctors and nurses who have been trained to proficiency in the skills to manage normal (uncomplicated) pregnancies, childbirth and the immediate postnatal period and to identify, manage or refer complications in the woman and newborn.' Source: WHO/ICM/FIGO Joint Statement on Skilled Attendant— Way Forward, forthcoming publication.

b   Given the low status of women, special emphasis is put on empowerment of women. The importance of the role of men as partners and fathers is recognized, but for purposes of this document, their role is considered as influential within household and community decision-making.

c   Skilled care is health care provided by a skilled attendant, backed up by the necessary systems and support required to enable them to function effectively and includes access to an effective referral system for emergency care for women and newborns with complications. See www.safemotherhood.org/resources/publications.html

d The additional benefits of a process of interaction (rather than being a passive recipient of information) and of taking external information and applying it within her own social and cultural context is further explained in the section on health education approaches. See also Santarelli[27], Young and Flower[11] and Sanders and Fitch[12].

e Also called birth planning, birth preparedness and complication readiness. It is noted that interventions developed in higher resource countries have focused on the psychological and physical comfort of women. Herein, the authors refer to interventions as they have generally been developed in lower-resource countries, focusing on measures to prepare for action in the event of obstetric emergencies and plan for the use of skilled care for birth.

f Moore[13] proposed the design, production and distribution of a 'birth preparedness card' to improve birth preparedness. The main objective of the card would be to improve household dialogue and compliance. Cards have been used in different programmes including CARE Bangladesh, Family Care International Skilled Care Initiative in Kenya and MotherCare Healthy Mother/Healthy Child Project in Egypt.

g It is noted that research on decision-making processes indicates that it may not be acceptable to project findings from studies in other health areas, as the setting may affect the decision-making process and, consequently, the outcomes[16].

h The JHPIEGO Maternal and Newborn Health (MNH) programme has developed a Birth Preparedness and Complication Readiness matrix which identifies the roles of the different stakeholders involved, including facilities and communities, policymakers, health care providers, families, and women. See http://www.mnh.jhpiego.org

i See JHPIEGO Maternal and Newborn Health (MNH) experience in Guatemala: http://www.mnh.jhpiego.org

j The process of creating knowledge is described in detail in Santarelli[27].

k The theoretical and implementation frameworks for this approach have been developed by IDEA—Institute for Development and Education of Adults. See Faundez[28] for more information on the PdT.

l Specific countries are: Brazil, Benin, Burkina Faso, Cape Verde, Colombia, Congo, El Salvador, Guatemala, Haiti, Jordan, Lebanon and Niger.

References

1 *Making Pregnancy Safer: Paper for Discussion*. Geneva: World Health Organization, 2000

2 *Health Promotion. Ottawa Charter*. Ottawa, Ontario, Canada (WHO/HPR/HEP/95.1). Geneva: World Health Organization, 1986

3 Santarelli C. *Working with Individuals, Families and Communities to Improve Maternal and Newborn Health*. Geneva: World Health Organization, 2003; In press

4 Gutzwiller F, Jeanneret O (eds). *Médecine social et préventive; Santé publique*. Berne: Editions Hans Huber, 1996

5 Aubel J. *Communication for Empowerment: Strengthening Partnerships for Community Health and Development*. New York: United Nations Children's Fund, 1999

6 *Choices in Family Planning: Informed and Voluntary Decision-making*. New York: Engenderhealth, 2003

7 World Health Organization, United Nations Children's Fund and United Nations Population Fund. *Women-friendly Health Services. Experiences in Maternal Care. Report of a WHO/UNICEF/UNFPA Workshop. Mexico City, Mexico, January 1999*. New York: United Nations Children's Fund, 1999

8 Kirkham M, Stapleton H (eds). *Informed Choice in Maternity Care: An Evaluation of Evidence-based Leaflets*. University of York, York: NHS Centre for Reviews and Disseminations, 2000

9 Murphy E, Steele C. Client–Provider Interactions in Family Planning Services: Guidance from research and program experience. *Recommendations for Updating Selected Practices in Contraceptive Use, Vol. II*. University of North Carolina, Chapel Hill: International Training in Health Program (INTRAH), December 1997

10 Kettunen T, Poskiparta M, Liimatainen L. Empowering counselling—a case study: nurse–patient encounter in a hospital. *Health Educ Res* 2001; **16**: 227–38

11   Young A, Flower L. Patients as partners, patients as problem-solvers. *Health Commun* 2002; **14**: 69–97

12   Sanders R, Fitch K. The actual practice of compliance seeking. *Commun Theory* 2001; **11**: 263–89

13   Moore KM. Safer Motherhood 2000: Toward a framework for behavior change to reduce maternal deaths. In: *The Communication Initiative, January 2000*, http://www.comminit.com/misc/safer_motherhood.html. Accessed on 23 May 2003

14   *Pregnancy, Childbirth, Post-partum and Newborn Care: An Essential Care Practice Guide.* Geneva: World Health Organization, 2003; In press

15   Elwyn G. *Shared Decision-Making: Patient Involvement in Clinical Practice.* University of Nijmegen, Nijmegen: Werkgroep Onderzoek Kwaliteit (WOK), 2001

16   Bekker H, Thornton JG, Airey CM *et al.* Informed decision-making: An annotated bibliography and systematic review. *Health Technol Assess* 1999; **3**

17   Charles CA, Whelan T, Gafni A *et al.* Shared treatment decision-making: what does it mean to physicians? *J Clin Oncol* 2003; **21**: 932–6

18   El Ansari W, Phillips CJ. Empowering healthcare workers in Africa: partnerships in health—beyond the rhetoric towards a model. *Crit Public Health* 2001; **11**: 231–51

19   Bravata DM, Rastegar A, Horwitz RI. How do women make decisions about hormone replacement therapy? *Am J Med* 2002; **113**: 22–9

20   Kim YM, Kols A, Bonnin C *et al.* Client communication behaviors with health care providers in Indonesia. *Patient Educ Couns* 2001; **45**: 59–68

21   O'Rourke K, Howard-Grabman L, Seoane G. Impact of community organization of women on perinatal outcomes in rural Bolivia. *Pan Am J Public Health* 1998; **3**: 9–14

22   Stetson V, Davis R. *Health Education in Primary HealthCare Projects: A Critical Review of Various Approaches.* Washington, DC: CORE Group/USAID, 1999. http://www.coregroup.org/resources/health_ed.pdf. Accessed on 20 April 2003

23   Waisbord S. *Family Tree of Theories: Methodologies and Strategies in Development Communication: Convergences and Differences.* New York: The Rockefeller Foundation, 2000. http://www.comminit.com/pdf/familytree.pdf. Accessed on 20 April 2003

24   Vygotski L. *Pensée et langage.* Paris: La Dispute, 1997

25   Bronckart JP. Semiotic interaction and cognitive construction. *Arch Psychol* 1997; **65**: 95–106

26   Sardan JPO. *Anthropologie et Développement.* Paris: Apad-Karthala, 1995

27   Santarelli C. *Behaviour Change, Social Change or Changing Ourselves.* Geneva: Enfants du Monde, 2002; draft document

28   Faundez A. The pedagogy of text briefly described. *Intercâmbios*, Institute for Development and Education of Adults 1999; **12**: 1

29   Cornwall A, Welborn A (eds). *Realizing Rights: Transforming Approaches to Sexual and Reproductive Well-being.* London: Zed Books, 2002

30   Kasaje DCO, Orinda V. *The Community Dialogue Model Based on the Principles of Partnership in Action for Health Focusing on Behaviour Change.* New York: United Nations Children's Fund, 2001

31   Howard-Grabman, L, Willis C, Quierolo C *et al.* A dialogue of knowledge approach to better reproductive, sexual and child health in rural Andean communities. In: Cornwall A, Welborn A (eds) *Realizing Rights: Transforming Approaches to Sexual and Reproductive Well-being.* London: Zed Books, 2002

32   El Ansari W, Phillips CJ, Zwi AB. Narrowing the gap between academic professional wisdom and community lay knowledge: perceptions from partnerships. *Public Health* 1992; **116**: 151–9

33   Gibbon M, Cazottes I. Working with women's groups to promote health in the community using the health analysis and action cycle within Nepal. *Qual Health Res* 2001; **11**: 728–50

34   Miller S, Sloan NL, Winkoff B *et al.* Where is the 'E' in MCH? The need for an evidence-based approach in safe motherhood. *J Midwifery Womens Health* 2003; **48**: 10–8

Promoting standards for quality of maternal health care

A Metin Gülmezoglu

HRP—UNDP/UNFPA/WHO/World Bank Special Programme on Research, Development and Research Training in Human Reproduction, Department of Reproductive Health and Research, World Health Organization, Geneva, Switzerland

Evidence-based health care with its emphasis on the need for searching, retrieving, summarizing and utilizing the best available evidence in decision-making has become essential in setting standards. Accordingly, maternity care standards should be based on best available evidence identified through systematic reviews of the literature. Promotion of standards relies on access to information, active strategies to facilitate professional behaviour change and efforts to sustain the change. Access to information is essential but insufficient to improve standards on its own. Changing professional behaviour is not accomplished easily. Active strategies based on the nature of the health care problem and an evaluation of the barriers that are likely to operate against change are required to influence professional behaviour. Once implemented, the standards should be regularly monitored and revised as new evidence becomes available.

Introduction

Correspondence to:
A Metin Gülmezoglu,
HRP—UNDP/UNFPA/WHO/
World Bank Special
Programme on Research,
Development and
Research Training in
Human Reproduction,
Department of
Reproductive Health and
Research, World Health
Organization, Avenue
Appia 20, Geneva 27,
CH-1211 Switzerland.
E-mail:
gulmezoglum@who.int

A variety of problems are caused when clinical practices that are not based on sound scientific evidence find their way into established medical/health care practice. It is generally acknowledged that removing an entrenched practice is much more difficult than introducing a new one. Thus, not only valuable resources continue to be used for practices of unknown effectiveness, but also, research is needed later to evaluate the usefulness of these practices. For example, large trials had to be conducted to show that routine episiotomy is not beneficial[1]. Furthermore, routine electronic fetal monitoring during labour[2], and routine ultrasound assessment during pregnancy[3], have not been shown to decrease morbidity and mortality. Yet these two practices are used widely in some developing countries. A more effective resource allocation, complemented by efforts to implement only those practices that are effective, should be a priority in order to improve the quality of maternity services in developing countries. Several steps are needed to improve and maintain high-quality care standards. Although the focus of this article is on clinical practices, the 'standards' should not be seen only within this context. The interpersonal dimensions of care and services are crucial to improving quality. This is especially relevant to reproductive health where the users of services are healthy women or couples in the majority of cases[4].

Pathways to improving standards

Access to information

A pre-requisite for need- and evidence-based allocation of resources and appropriate health care practices is to have access to scientifically solid and up-to-date information. Without access to information, it is extremely difficult to maintain or improve the quality of care, which places a further burden on the limited resources for health care in developing countries as ineffective and/or harmful practices remain in practice.

Most health workers and policy-makers in developing countries do not have easy access to the latest reliable information on effective care. This is not only because of the high cost and erratic delivery of most subscription journals, but also because few medical journals publish comprehensive systematic reviews on the effectiveness of health care interventions in developing countries. Such information remains scattered in different papers in numerous journals, making it very difficult for health practitioners to get a good overview of all the data available on a given subject.

The challenge therefore is to develop a strategy to provide access to good quality and up-to-date information. Furthermore, the information provided should be comprehensive enough to reduce the need for additional information to guide decision-making. *The WHO Reproductive Health Library* (RHL) is a collaborative effort between the World Health Organization, the Cochrane Collaboration and scientists in developing countries that attempts to meet this challenge[5]. RHL includes Cochrane systematic reviews in all areas of reproductive health with commentaries from individuals with knowledge of the typical settings in low-income countries. RHL is available to health workers on a free subscription in low- and middle-income countries and its contents are updated and expanded on an annual basis. The free subscription system and the assistance of WHO collaborating institutions worldwide provide RHL access to more than 30,000 health workers every year. The CD-ROM format enables annual updates and revisions as and when new evidence becomes available. Furthermore, RHL includes tools such as implementation manuals, video clips and slide shows to facilitate the adoption of evidence-based practices.

Another recently initiated project is the Health Internetwork (HINARI)[6]. This project coordinated by the World Health Organization provides access to the Internet versions of the main health care journals (around 2000 journals) free or at very low prices in low-income countries. Notwithstanding the difficulties of poor quality telephone lines and Internet access costs, the project is important in bringing the major publishers together for the purpose of providing access to information[7].

Innovative approaches are required to reach health workers in low-income countries efficiently. The developments in information technology provide more opportunities. For example, The Health Channel launched by the Interactive Health Network and WorldSpace aims to provide information to lay public and health workers through radio and data casting using satellite technology[8]. Although the effectiveness of such approaches remains to be seen, it seems worthwhile to explore alternative routes.

Facilitating behaviour change and establishing the standards

The objective of accessing information is to keep up-to-date and change practices that are ineffective or harmful in favour of those that have been demonstrated to be more effective by rigorous research methods.

However, although access to information is crucial, it is rarely sufficient on its own to lead to change. Improving or changing clinical practice with the availability of new knowledge is a complex and often difficult process. These difficulties are increasingly recognized. The new knowledge needs to be assessed taking into consideration the socio-cultural and economic contexts. Even when there is general acceptance of a new treatment, there may be barriers to overcome. Grol et al[9] outlined attributes of practice guidelines that make them more or less amenable to adoption. The guidelines that were on controversial issues, including change in daily routines, and that were vague were less likely to be implemented. Even for those practices that are clear, non-controversial and do not require major changes in daily work, some additional measures are required to implement the practice within a given period of time[10]. It must be acknowledged that adoption of new practices almost always involves trade-offs. These trade-offs may relate to beneficial effects versus side-effects or to socio-cultural and economic contexts[11].

Planned dissemination and implementation strategies using appropriate tools for appropriate target populations are necessary to bring improvements in standards of care. Several different strategies exist alone or in combination, based on different theories of behavioural change. Of these, continued educational meetings in the form of interactive workshops seem to have moderate effects in improving practice[12].

Educational outreach, targeting local opinion leaders, reminders and audit and feedback are some of the strategies that have been used with varying degrees of success. More evidence on implementation strategies can be found in several systematic reviews published in the *Cochrane Library* by the Cochrane Effective Practice and Organization of Care Group[13].

Best practices are selected from those that have been shown to have more benefit than harm according to the results of systematic reviews. In a similar way, principles of evidence-based health care should be followed when selecting the strategy for implementing the best practices as shown in Figure 1. The assessment of the barriers is an essential step to guide the selection of the strategy for implementing change. There may be fewer or easier barriers to overcome to change some practices while others may be more complex. It must be remembered that it may not be possible or feasible to elucidate all potential barriers upfront. For example, changing from one type of uterotonic (ergometrine) to another (oxytocin) would be expected to be relatively straightforward if the agent is available (although a new procurement policy may not be that easy to generalize in a bureaucratic setting). Using oxytocin instead of ergometrine for the management of the third stage of labour would not require changes in daily routine, learning new procedures or cost more. However, the implementation of a programme of labour companionship to reduce obstetric interventions and increase maternal satisfaction with care is likely to be more complex. The facilities may lack sufficient privacy, the staff may not be too keen on having other non-professional people around, the labour companions may need training, and there

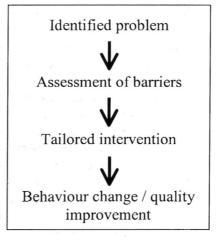

Fig. 1 Tailoring interventions to improve standards.

may be some costs and other unforeseen barriers. The process outlined in Figure 1 can be useful to facilitate the change. It is important to consciously assess the barriers because the design (or the target) of the intervention to establish the change will be based on overcoming those particular barriers.

Another important concern is to maintain the standards once the change has been accomplished. In this respect, clinical audit could be an important tool. Clinical audit is a useful strategy to improve the clinical care alone, although the effect size could be modest[14].

Some locally developed implementation projects using evidence-based strategies exist. The Better Births Initiative is a collaborative project attempting to improve and maintain standards of care during labour and childbirth[15]. This project involves educational workshops in maternity wards focusing on evidence-based and humane practices concerning the care of women during labour and childbirth. An audit programme is also proposed as part of the workshops so that the staff can monitor the standards of care themselves.

Best practices in maternal health care

The WHO Programme To Map Best Reproductive Health Practices[16] together with the Cochrane Collaboration and other partner institutions develop and maintain systematic reviews of reproductive health practices that are especially relevant to low-income countries. These practices are included in RHL together with tools to facilitate their incorporation into services. Some of the important practices are listed in Tables 1–6 according to their level of effectiveness. These tables are included in RHL to provide a snapshot of effectiveness of practices and are also linked to the evidence supporting those statements.

Table 1 Beneficial forms of care

- Active management of the third stage of labour on decreasing blood loss after delivery

- Antibiotics for preterm prelabour rupture of membranes prolong pregnancy and reduce maternal and infant infectious morbidity

- Antibiotic prophylaxis for women undergoing caesarean section reduces postoperative infectious complications

- Antibiotic treatment of asymptomatic bacteriuria prevents pyelonephritis in pregnancy and reduces preterm delivery

- Corticosteroids prior to preterm delivery reduce neonatal mortality, respiratory distress syndrome and intraventricular haemorrhage

- External cephalic version at term reduces breech delivery and caesarean section rates

(Continued on next page)

Table 1 (continued) Beneficial forms of care

- Intraumbilical vein injection of saline solution with oxytocin reduces the need for manual removal of placenta

- Magnesium sulphate therapy for women with eclampsia is more effective in preventing further fits than other anticonvulsants

- Magnesium sulphate therapy for women with pre-eclampsia reduces eclampsia and maternal deaths

- Nevirapine given intrapartum followed by a single dose to the newborn within 72 h reduces the risk of mother-to-child transmission of HIV infection

- Population-based iodine supplementation in severely iodine deficient areas prevents cretinism and infant deaths due to iodine deficiency

- Reduced number of antenatal care visits with specific activities compared to higher number of visits in standard western style antenatal care costs less without an increase in adverse outcomes

- Routine early pregnancy ultrasound improves the accuracy of gestational age determination and reduces the need for labour induction for postterm pregnancy

- Routine induction of labour after 41 completed weeks reduces perinatal death, caesarean section and meconium stained amniotic fluid

- Routine iron and folate supplementation during pregnancy prevent maternal anaemia at delivery or 6 weeks postpartum

- Routine midwife/general practitioner led antenatal care for low-risk women, compared to specialist led care, costs less without an increase in adverse outcomes

- Routine periconceptional folate supplementation reduces the occurrence of neural tube defects and their recurrence

- Social support during labour in busy, technology-oriented settings reduces the need for pain relief and is associated with a positive labour experience

- Syphilis screening and treatment decreases the incidence of congenital syphilis

- Zidovudine given as long or short course reduces the risk of mother-to-child transmission of HIV infection

Table 2 Forms of care likely to be beneficial

- Antimalarial prophylaxis or presumptive treatment during pregnancy to primigravidae in endemic malarious areas increases birth weight and decreases the incidence of low-birth-weight babies

- Antimalarial prophylaxis or presumptive treatment during pregnancy in endemic malarious areas decreases subsequent fever and sickness episodes

- Antimalarial prophylaxis during pregnancy in endemic malarious areas reduces subsequent fever and sickness episodes

- Antimalarial prophylaxis or presumptive treatment during pregnancy in endemic malarious areas reduces the incidence of maternal anaemia in late pregnancy

- Balanced protein/energy supplementation during pregnancy to women with malnutrition or low calorie intake reduces the number of low-birth-weight babies and increases birth weight

- Breast and nipple stimulation at term is likely to reduce the incidence of post-term pregnancy

(Continued on next page)

Table 2 (continued from opposite page)

- Calcium supplementation to nulliparous women living in low-calcium intake areas reduces the rate of pre-eclampsia

- Exclusive breastfeeding up to 6 months reduces morbidity and possibly mortality due to diarrhoeal infections

- Genital chlamydia infection treatment with erythromycin or amoxycillin during pregnancy to achieve microbiological cure

- Gonorrhoea treatment during pregnancy with broad-spectrum antibiotics in low penicillinase-producing-*Neisseria gonorrhoeae* (PPNG) areas to achieve microbiological cure

- Kangaroo-mother care method of skin-to-skin contact in low-birth-weight infants is associated with reduced likelihood of illness at 6 months and exclusive breastfeeding at discharge from hospital

- Routine early pregnancy ultrasound by experienced staff is likely to be effective for early detection of fetal abnormalities and multiple pregnancies

- Social support during labour in busy, technology-oriented settings could lower caesarean section rates, lower number of infants with low Apgar scores (< 7 at 5 min) and lower duration of labour

- Vitamin A supplementation to very-low-birth-weight infants may reduce death and oxygen-treatment at 1 month of age

Table 3 Forms of care with a trade-off

- Amnioinfusion during labour for treatment of cord compression is effective in correcting fetal heart rate (FHR) abnormalities, Apgar scores (fewer babies with low Apgar), birth asphyxia and lowering caesarean section rates (when indication for caesarean section is based on FHR criteria alone), but safety of amnioinfusion concerning rare but serious maternal complications is not established

- Amnioinfusion during labour when moderate or thick meconium is noted is effective in reducing the incidence of meconium below cords, meconium aspiration syndrome and lowering caesarean section rate, but safety of amnioinfusion concerning rare but serious maternal complications is not established

- Antihypertensive therapy for mild to moderate hypertension during pregnancy is effective in reducing the incidence of severe hypertension. Beta-blockers are associated with fewer cases of proteinuria/pre-eclampsia but more small-for-gestational age babies

- Antiplatelet agents are associated with a 15% reduction in the incidence of pre-eclampsia. However, between 59 and 167 women need to be given antiplatelets to prevent one case of pre-eclampsia

- As part of active management of the third stage of labour, ergot preparations, compared to oxytocin, are more effective in reducing blood loss but are associated with smaller but significant increases in blood pressure, nausea and vomiting

- Gentamicin–clindamycin combination is the most effective antibiotic regimen for the treatment of endometritis after delivery. However, affordability may be a problem with clindamycin

- Intramuscular prostaglandins are effective in reducing blood loss in the third stage of labour but their safety is uncertain and their costs are prohibitive in under-resourced settings

- Planned caesarean section is overall significantly beneficial for the baby. In settings with high perinatal mortality these benefits are not as clear. The impact of large-scale implementation of a policy of caesarean section in terms of capability of performing vaginal breech delivery as an emergency procedure and the fate of women with previous caesarean section in areas where access is problematic is unknown

(Continued on next page)

Table 3 (continued) Forms of care with a trade-off

- Vaginal misoprostol administration for induction of labour in doses of 25 μg 3 hourly or more is more effective than oxytocin or other prostaglandins but it is associated with increased FHR abnormalities and uterine hyperstimulation. Vaginal misoprostol in doses of 25 μg 4–6 hourly is likely to be less effective but safer in terms of FHR abnormalities and uterine hyperstimulation

- When compared to intermittent auscultation of the heart rate, routine electronic FHR monitoring during labour is associated with fewer neonatal seizures, similar long-term infant outcome, but increased caesarean section rates

Table 4 Forms of care of unknown effectiveness

- Amnioinfusion during labour to correct cord compression on caesarean section rates when decision is based on not only fetal heart rate (FHR) monitoring criteria but also scalp blood gas analyses

- Amnioinfusion for moderate or thick meconium staining during labour on reducing perinatal mortality due to meconium aspiration

- Antimalarial prophylaxis during pregnancy in endemic malarious areas on preterm delivery and perinatal mortality

- Balanced protein/energy supplementation during pregnancy to women with malnutrition or low calorie intake on reducing preterm delivery, perinatal mortality and improving long-term neurocognitive development

- Complex fetal monitoring using computerized cardiotocography, amniotic fluid index and other biophysical profile measurements to improve the outcome of postterm pregnancies

- Ideal treatment of iron deficiency anaemia during pregnancy with iron tablets, parenteral iron or blood transfusion according to the level of anaemia

- Nutritional advice during pregnancy to improve maternal and infant outcomes

- Routine symphysis–fundal height measurements during pregnancy to detect impaired fetal growth and prevent perinatal mortality

- Using postural manoeuvres to convert breech to vertex presentation on incidence of breech delivery

- Antimicrobial therapy for gonorrhoea and genital chlamydia during pregnancy on the prevention of ophthalmia neonatorum

- Mass treatment of all community members for sexually transmitted infections

- Metronidazole treatment of asymptomatic trichomoniasis to reduce adverse pregnancy outcomes such as preterm birth

- Screening and treatment for bacterial vaginosis to reduce the preterm delivery rate

- Routine topical antiseptic or antibiotic application to the umbilical cord to prevent sepsis and other illness in the neonate

- The effectiveness of kangaroo-mother care method in reducing neonatal and infant mortality and exclusive breastfeeding at 1 or 6 months is unknown

Table 5 Forms of care likely to be ineffective

- Antibiotics in preterm labour with intact membranes to prolong pregnancy and reduce preterm birth
- Anticonvulsants in full-term newborns with perinatal asphyxia for preventing mortality and morbidity
- Early amniotomy during labour in reducing caesarean section rates
- External cephalic version before term to reduce the incidence of breech presentation at delivery
- Isocaloric protein supplementation during pregnancy to improve pregnancy outcomes
- Ketanserin for rapid lowering of very high blood pressure during pregnancy
- Oral or rectal misoprostol as part of active management of the third stage of labour for the prevention of postpartum haemorrhage
- Routine early pregnancy ultrasound in decreasing perinatal mortality
- Routine electronic fetal monitoring during labour for low-risk pregnancies
- Routine intubation at birth in vigorous term meconium-stained babies to prevent meconium aspiration syndrome
- Social support during the course of pregnancy before labour in improving biological pregnancy outcomes and mothers' satisfaction

Table 6 Forms of care likely to be harmful

- A policy of routine episiotomy to prevent perineal/vaginal tears compared to restricted use of episiotomy
- Diazoxide for rapid lowering of severe high blood pressure during pregnancy because of severe hypotension
- Forceps extraction instead of vacuum extraction for assisted vaginal delivery when both are applicable is associated with increased incidence of trauma to the maternal genital tract
- Using diazepam, phenytoin and lytic cocktail to prevent further fits in women with eclampsia when magnesium sulphate is available

The practices listed in Tables 1 and 2 indicate those that are more likely to have benefits than harm. It should be noted that these practices vary according to the outcomes. That is, an intervention may be beneficial in preventing an adverse outcome but may be ineffective for another. Similarly, for some practices, in addition to the benefits, there may be a possibility of harm (Table 3). The decision then depends on the trade-offs and how acceptable those are to individual women and to the communities.

There are some pregnancy pathologies for which our understanding of the pathophysiology is poor and the preventive or therapeutic interventions are either non-existent or weak. Pre-eclampsia/eclampsia and preterm birth are good examples. However, there are many interventions where strong evidence exists regarding effectiveness and these should be transferred to services as a matter of urgency. We do not have an effective preventive strategy for pre-eclampsia but we have magnesium sulphate to prevent eclampsia and reduce further convulsions in women who have experienced eclamptic convulsions. Another concern in the field of pregnancy and childbirth is the removal of practices that are ineffective or harmful (Tables 5 and 6). Unfortunately, practices implemented following logical arguments decades ago remain entrenched even if there is compelling evidence against them.

Conclusions

During the past decades, significant developments in health care research methodologies, health care provision and programme development have been taking place. The nature of information dissemination, access and utilization is also rapidly changing. Innovative strategies to disseminate and improve access to information are necessary to keep up with the pace of development in the twenty-first century. Evidence-based health care with its emphasis on utilizing the best available evidence in decision-making is here to stay. Consequently, clinicians and policy-makers need to be familiar with concepts such as search strategies, critical appraisal and meta-analysis. Maintaining standards increasingly requires interdisciplinary collaboration among doctors, midwives, librarians, statisticians and other health professionals. Evidence-based health care practice should be complemented by evidence-based implementation strategies.

References

1 Argentine Episiotomy Trial Collaborative Group. Routine vs selective episiotomy: a randomised controlled trial. *Lancet* 1993; **342**: 1517–8
2 Thacker SB, Stroup D, Chang M. Continuous electronic heart rate monitoring for fetal assessment during labor (Cochrane Review). In: *The Cochrane Library, Issue 2, 2003*. Oxford: Update Software
3 Neilson JP. Ultrasound for fetal assessment in early pregnancy (Cochrane Review). In: *The Cochrane Library, Issue 2,* 2003. Oxford: Update Software
4 Bruce J. Fundamental elements of quality of care. *Stud Fam Plann* 1990; **21**: 61–91
5 WHO Reproductive Health Library, No. 6. Geneva: World Health Organization, 2003 (WHO/RHR/03.5)
6 Health Internetwork. http://www.healthinternetwork.org/index.php?lang=en (accessed 27 May 2003)
7 Smith R. Closing the digital divide. *BMJ* 2003; **326**: 238
8 Interactive Health Network. http://www.ihn.info (accessed 01 June 2003)
9 Grol R, Dalhuijsen J, Thomas S, Veld C, Rutten G, Mokkink H. Attributes of clinical guidelines that influence use of guidelines in general practice: observational study. *BMJ* 1998; **317**: 858–61
10 EBHC. Getting evidence into practice. *Effective Health Care* 1999; **5**: 1–16
11 Irwig L, Zwarenstein M, Zwi A, Chalmers I. A flow diagram to facilitate selection of interventions and research for health care. *Bull World Health Organ* 1998; **76**: 17–24

12   Thomson O'Brien MA, Freemantle N, Oxman AD, Wolf F, Davis DA, Herrin J. Continuing education meetings and workshops: effects on professional practice and health care outcomes (Cochrane Review). In: *The Cochrane Library, Issue 1, 2003*. Oxford: Update Software

13   Effective Practice and Organization of Care Group. http://www.epoc.uottawa.ca/ (accessed 02 June 2003)

14   Thomson O'Brien MA, Oxman AD, Davis DA, Haynes RB, Freemantle N, Harvey EL. Audit and feedback versus alternative strategies: effects on professional practice and health care outcomes (Cochrane Review). In: *The Cochrane Library, Issue 1, 2003*. Oxford: Update Software

15   Better Births Initiative. http://www.liv.ac.uk/lstm/bbimainpage.html (accessed 27 May 2003)

16   The WHO Programme To Map Best Reproductive Health Practices. http://www.who.int/reproductive-health/rhl/index.html (accessed 02 June 2003)

Pregnancy—reducing maternal deaths and disability in Sri Lanka: national strategies

Dulitha Fernando*, Anoma Jayatilleka† and Vinitha Karunaratna†

*Faculty of Medicine, University of Colombo and †Family Health Bureau, Ministry of Health, Colombo, Sri Lanka

The declining trend in the maternal mortality rate (MMR) from the 1930s to the late 1990s resulted from several strategies implemented within and outside the health sector. Expansion of both field-based and institutional services through the past decades contributed to improved geographical access and provision of 'free' services improved economic access. These led to increased use of antenatal and natal services provided by trained midwives and other personnel followed by improvements in the availability of specialized care and emergency obstetric care. Integration of family planning and other inputs to the maternal health programme has yielded positive results. The role of the private sector is limited to provision of a component of antenatal services. The organization for service provision and an information system made significant contributions towards improvement. The commitment of the health sector to provide services free of charge supported by non-health inputs, especially female education, has enabled Sri Lanka to make gains in maternal health.

Introduction

Sri Lanka is an island in the Indian ocean with a population of 18.7 million[1] spread over a land area of 62,705 square kilometres. Currently, a country with a parliamentary democratic system of government, Sri Lanka was under colonial rule during the period 1505–1948, first under Portuguese rule, then Dutch followed by British, who colonized the whole country. In 1931, some degree of autonomy was given to the nationals under the Donoughmore constitution, until the country became independent in 1948.

Sri Lanka is often considered as a low income country with a per capita GNP of US\$ 823 in 2002[2] and with relatively good health indicators, a maternal mortality rate (MMR) of 0.23 and an infant mortality rate (IMR) of 16.3 per 1000 live births in 1996. The life expectancy for females is higher, 75.4 years compared with 70.7 years for males for the period 1996–2001, and the literacy level is comparatively high (90.1%)

Correspondence to:
Prof. Dulitha Fernando,
Department of
Community Medicine,
Faculty of Medicine,
University of Colombo,
Kynsey Road, Colombo 8,
Sri Lanka.
E-mail: sunithf@sltnet.lk

compared with the other countries of the region, with female literacy being 87.9%[3].

Development of maternal health services—historical background

Development of specific services for mothers in Sri Lanka can be traced back to ancient and medieval times. According to ancient chronicles, the first maternity home was probably established between 522 and 524 AD[4].

The Portuguese introduced the western system of medical care to the country in 1505. The Dutch, who ruled the country from 1658 to 1796, established a few hospitals in the Maritime Provinces. The present day health services of Sri Lanka aimed at provision of the 'western' system of medicine evolved from the military and estate medical services introduced by the British, during the period when they ruled Sri Lanka.

The earliest indication of a health service aimed specifically at mothers and children was the establishment of a Maternity Hospital in 1897. The next recorded maternal and child health activity was the setting up of a Public Health Department in the Colombo Municipal Council in 1902 and the establishment of a Maternal and Child Health (MCH) Department in 1906. In 1927, the midwifery services in the Colombo Municipality were re-organized by training all midwives working in the Municipality.

The inauguration of the Donoughmore Commission in 1931, with a Minister in charge of all health services, gave a new impetus to all activities related to health services. At this time, the prevailing health situation showed a high incidence of communicable diseases and poor health standards, with a MMR of 20.3 and IMR of 176 per 1000 live births. The periodic census carried out provided data related to population, which enabled an assessment of some indicators on maternal and child health status.

By this time, Sri Lanka had experience of the positive economic impact of a preventive programme aimed at the community, clearly demonstrated with the helminthiasis control programme. This led to the establishment of a 'Health Unit' on an experimental basis in 1926, emphasizing preventive and promotive health activities aimed at the community level. A team of field level health workers working with a Medical Officer carried out the activities, which included provision of maternal and child care at community level.

A health unit could be described as a defined geographical area, hence with a defined population, under a Medical Officer of Health (MOH). Several categories of health workers work as a team with the MOH, namely the Public Health Nurse (PHN), Public Health Inspector (PHI) and Public Health Midwife (PHM). The MCH services were to be provided at domiciliary level and at clinics established at 'health centres' (field level service outlets), within the health unit area. The PHM was responsible for antenatal, natal and postnatal services.

The Medical Ordinance of 1927 made provisions for registration of midwives, which was made a legal requirement. The enactment requiring compulsory registration of births and deaths enacted in 1897 provided data from these registrations which could be used to assess problems related to maternal and child mortality. By 1931, the provisions in the Medical Ordinance referring to the registration of midwives were enforced only in the Colombo Municipality.

Trends in maternal mortality

In 1931, the available indicators on maternal and child health were far from satisfactory—a MMR of 21.4 and an IMR of 175 per 1000 live births. Changes in the MMR between 1931 and 1947 (pre-independence era) show a declining trend, except for the sharp increase in 1935 to 26.5, attributed to the malaria epidemic which led to high mortality in all age groups (Fig. 1).

An effective control programme with DDT spraying brought the situation under control[5]. Other than this unusual occurrence, the decline continued until 1947, when the MMR was approximately 50% of that in 1931.

During the early post-independence period, from 1948 up to 1960, the decline in MMR continued, from 6.3 in 1948 to 3.4 in 1960, *i.e.* a 46% decline. The next 15 years from 1962 to 1977 saw a more marked decline, 3.0 in 1962 to 0.8 for 1977, and a further reduction occurred in the years that followed.

Leading causes of maternal deaths varied (Table 1). During the period 1931–1947, sepsis and convulsions were the leading causes of death, with haemorrhages being next in order of importance. In the early 1950s, toxaemia of pregnancy became the leading cause and by the mid-1960s, haemorrhages of pregnancy and childbirth were the most important cause of maternal deaths, with anaemia, sepsis and toxaemia being the other major causes[6]. In recent decades, the important contribution made by deaths due to abortions and attributed to 'other causes' has shown an upward trend.

National level strategies for reduction in maternal mortality and disability

When Sri Lanka gained independence in February 1948, several social welfare schemes that included food subsidies, free education system,

Trends in Maternal Mortality 1931-1996

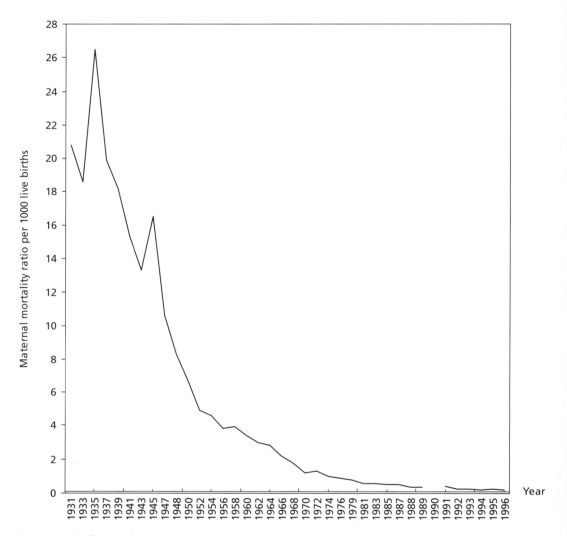

Fig. 1 Trend of MMR during the period 1931–1996.

food supplementation and a health service provided free of charge were available and continued after independence. The Department of Medical Services established before independence was responsible for planning and implementing health services in the state sector.

Over the past seven decades, several strategies were adopted by the health sector and by other sectors that contributed to the lowering of maternal mortality, with morbidity and disability gaining attention in recent years.

Table 1 Percentage contribution made by selected causes, to maternal mortality, 1930–2000

Year	Abortion	Sepsis	Haemorrhage	PIH	Other	Total
1930	0.82	36.45	2.94	47.27	12.51	100.00
1935	0.89	32.51	3.14	50.01	13.46	100.00
1940	1.56	29.76	7.00	47.25	14.53	100.10
1945	1.34	24.55	8.24	46.19	19.68	100.00
1950	1.47	20.15	21.39	28.72	28.07	99.82
1955	2.88	17.66	22.52	30.48	26.46	100.00
1960	2.74	11.43	28.79	24.77	32.27	100.00
1965	2.38	9.73	28.39	26.92	32.58	100.00
1970	6.17	13.46	30.65	25.42	24.30	100.00
1975	6.23	6.23	33.25	28.05	26.23	100.00
1980	10.74	4.81	18.52	35.56	30.37	100.00
1985	11.17	3.05	31.47	23.86	30.46	100.00
1991	11.26	1.32	43.05	18.54	25.83	100.00
1995	17.28	1.23	48.15	3.70	29.63	100.00
1996	6.25	1.25	35.00	2.50	55.00	100.00
1999[a]	8.69	4.89	20.11	12.50	53.80	99.99
2000[a]	13.22	4.76	19.57	7.40	55.02	99.97

Sources: Reports from the Registrar General's Department.
[a]Data from the Family Health Bureau, Ministry of Health.

Expansion of facilities for service provision

Field health services

The initiative taken in 1926 to provide field-based health services though a system of health units was continued, so that by 1952 the health unit areas covered the entire country and the role of the untrained midwife at the village level diminished. With the available evidence pointing to the positive contribution made by the health units to reduction in MMR in the early years of its implementation, two important policy decisions were taken to improve the MCH services. They were the introduction of health education as a component of such services and the integration of MCH services with other activities carried out in health units, *e.g.* sanitation, prevention of communicable diseases[7].

Institutional health facilities

These were developed throughout the island, leading to the establishment of a network of institutions ranging from General Hospitals at the highest level to Rural Hospitals at the lowest. Thus, the number of state sector hospitals increased from 112 in 1931 to 263 in 1955[8].

Facilities available at the institutions were improved with access to specialized services in the higher level of hospitals, which served as referral centres. This strategy enabled easier geographical access to services and provision of services free of charge enabled economic access. Availability of a satisfactory road network enhanced the accessibility. In addition to the institutions of the Department of Health Services available for deliveries, several local authorities, especially the Municipalities, provided Maternity Homes, where deliveries were attended to by trained midwives[9].

The high levels of maternal mortality reported in the pre-independence years, *i.e.* 1931–1947, were mainly due to sepsis and convulsions which contributed to approximately 84% of all maternal deaths, indicating the need for skilled antenatal care and trained assistance at childbirth[10].

Provision of antenatal care

During the late pre- and early post-independence periods, antenatal services through clinics held at government institutions continued along with the expansion of the health unit system to provide domiciliary services for pregnant women by trained field midwives and antenatal clinics held in 'health centres' in health units.

Improving availability of skilled attendance at birth

This was a key strategy adopted through both expansion of the health unit system which provided assistance from trained midwives in home-based deliveries and by increasing the availability of facilities for institutional deliveries. By 1958, about 58% of the births were attended to by skilled personnel, of which 25% were deliveries in the home. The percentage of institutional deliveries showed a sharp upward trend in the decades that followed, increasing to 92% of all deliveries taking place in institutions in the year 2001[11].

To have a positive impact on the outcome, the expansion of services to improve antenatal and natal care has to be linked with adequate utilization of the services provided. This point is clearly made by the Director General of the Department of Medical Services in his reports in the mid-1940s where he states that 'there has been an encouraging demand from the public for improved facilities for maternal care, not only in Colombo but throughout the island specially in rural areas'[12].

Enforcement of legal enactments that necessitated registration of midwives

This was expanded to areas outside Colombo. Registration of vital statistical data was continued and formed the basis on which the services could be evaluated.

With further decline in the MMR and with haemorrhages of pregnancy becoming important causes of maternal mortality, it became necessary to adopt strategies that would address these needs. Development and expansion of the facilities for blood transfusion took place during the late 1950s and 1960s[13]. In addition, PHMs were trained to administer ergometrine orally, and PHNs and nurses in smaller hospitals were allowed to give ergometrine parenterally.

By 1959, with a lower MMR, the importance of maternal morbidity was emphasized. Proper antenatal care for early detection of toxaemia and programmes for the prevention of anaemia were considered important and given emphasis accordingly.

Family planning

The family planning (FP) programme was gradually integrated into the MCH services of the Department of Health Services, and the services were provided by the personnel of the Department of Health, mainly through the MOH and field staff.

Family planning activities became an integral part of the services provided by the state sector by 1965 and this led to a well organized family planning service throughout the country which included counselling services, sale of contraceptives at field level, provision of other services (IUCD insertions, DMPA injections) at field level clinics and facilities for sterilization (both males and females) at different levels of institutions. Data from the Demographic and Health Surveys conducted in 1987, 1993 and 2000 show a consistent upward trend in contraceptive prevalence rates: 55% in 1987, 61% in 1993 and 70% in 2000[14–16].

Training of personnel

Several categories of personnel were required for the provision of services outlined above. They included medical officers, PHNs, midwives and other relevant categories in the curative institutions. Medical Officers were trained at the Ceylon Medical College, established in 1870. With the establishment of the University of Ceylon, the Medical College became the Faculty of Medicine of the University in 1942. Facilities for training of Medical Officers expanded with the establishment of a second medical school in 1960 and four more medical schools in the next few decades.

Training of midwives commenced in two centres in 1931, the duration of training being 18 months. By 1947, the number of such training centres had increased to six. Training of PHNs was conducted at the Health Unit at Kalutara. The number of training institutes for nurses and midwives increased within the next two decades and the facilities for field training of the PHNs and PHMs at the 'Institute of Hygiene' at Kalutara were improved. The number of posts in categories concerned with the provision of preventive health services was increased gradually.

Establishment of postgraduate medical education in Sri Lanka in the mid-1970s is yet another important aspect of human resource development. All training programmes were funded entirely by the state.

Organization of the maternal care programme

Availability of an organizational structure for provision of maternal health services at the time of independence and the political commitment at the highest level for implementation of welfare measures were crucial factors that influenced the programme aimed at improving maternal health.

State sector

By 1960, the state sector health services responsible for the major component of the maternal care services identified the need for development of appropriate policies and programmes to further improve the situation. Following the recommendations of a committee appointed to re-organize the HCH services, a full time Medical Officer (MCH) was appointed in 1961 to intensify MCH work and a maternal and child health advisory committee under the chairmanship of the Deputy Director of Public Health Services. A special committee to investigate all maternal deaths was appointed in 1960 and a data collection form to be used in this investigation was developed.

In the next few decades, with the changing needs and emphasis on a wider scope for prevention of maternal mortality and disability, changes were made in the organizational structure for provision of maternal care. These included the establishment of the Family Planning Bureau in 1965, followed by the appointment of an Assistant Director, MCH to be in charge of MCH activities including family planning, 2 years later. In 1972, following the integration of the organization of MCH services with the FP services at the policy making level, the Family Health Bureau was established. In recent years, emphasis has been placed on increasing the availability of specialist services and for improved provision of facilities for emergency obstetric care.

Private sector

Though there are no data on the contribution made by the private sector to maternal health services, it can be assumed that their main contribution is in the provision of antenatal care. The Demographic and Health Survey of 2000 reports that in the year 2000, 5.5% of all deliveries took place in private hospitals[16].

Information system

Introduction of a system for registration of births and deaths as early as 1897 was the first step in the development of an information system. In the early post-independence era, such information formed the basis on which service requirements were identified, planned and implemented.

With further development of MCH services, data collection systems for monitoring the services were developed, based on the needs. Introduction of a comprehensive MCH/FP information system in 1986 enabled data from field level MCH activities to be assessed. This system has been further revised in the year 2000, to include information on the wide range of activities included under the family health programme, focusing on mothers and young children.

Completeness of registration of births and deaths has been considered to be satisfactory[17]. However, several circumstances have led to a deterioration of coverage of maternal deaths[18]. In recent years, alternative approaches were used to collect data on maternal deaths, through reports from field staff and from institutions. Maternal deaths were made notifiable in 1989. Maternal death investigations have been carried out since 1989. MMR for the year 2000, calculated on the basis of such reporting, was 57 per 100,000 live births, indicating under-reporting[19].

International organizations

The contribution by international organizations towards the national strategies ranged from support for development of physical facilities, provision of supplies and equipment to supporting training programmes locally and overseas and consultancy services. All funds available for maternal health activities are channelled though the Family Health Bureau of the Ministry of Health.

Non-governmental organizations (NGOs)

The role of NGOs in MCH activities was through provision of services and/or by assisting in community mobilization programmes and other support programmes for improvement of maternal care.

Contributions made by the programmes outside the health sector

In Sri Lanka, there were several welfare programmes that existed at the time of independence. Some of these programmes have been considered to have made a major contribution to the success of the programmes implemented through the health sector.

Educational reforms

With the introduction of Educational Ordinance of 1939 and the reforms that came into effect in the early 1940s, a free education system was gradually introduced on a national scale, affording equal opportunities for both males and females. The introduction of the free education system is considered to have had a long-term beneficial effect on the health status at national level, especially for the health of mothers and children. It has been suggested that the empowerment of women and education have been two key factors that have influenced the utilization of health services which contributed to the decline in the MMR[20].

Food subsidies

The Food Commissioner's Department set up in 1942 was given the task of distributing 2.5 pounds of rice per week per person at subsidized rates. This scheme, though not specifically targeted to mothers and children, could be considered to have had an impact on the MCH status by ensuring availability of a proportion of the nutrient requirement to a given family, especially during the war years. The food subsidy scheme underwent many changes in subsequent decades and has minimal inputs at the present time.

Food supplementation programmes

One of the earliest food supplementation programmes was the milk feeding scheme aimed at improving the nutritional status of pregnant women and pre-school children, introduced in the mid-1940s, by the Food Commissioner's Department in collaboration with the Department of Medical Services. During the past four decades, the ongoing programme has been the Thriposha programme implemented through the health services, whereby a food supplement based on corn and soya is provided to pregnant and lactating women.

Maternity Benefits Ordinance

The Maternity Benefit Ordinance No. 32 of 1939 enabled all employed women except casual employees to have access to maternity benefits: mainly maternity leave on pay for 6 weeks. Amendments to this ordinance in 1946 and 1952 revised the period of employment which entitled an employed woman to the above benefits. Further amendments made in 1978 and 1986 were mainly for the benefit of the infant and the young child.

Current status of maternal health and maternal health services

In spite of major changes in the economic policies, the government of Sri Lanka continued to provide a health service to the population, free of charge and training of all health personnel required for the services in the state sector has been under the free education system. Some of the key indicators related to maternal health as of 2001 are given in Table 2.

The Family Health Bureau is responsible for planning, co-ordinating, monitoring and evaluating the programme provision of family health services through the health infrastructure of the Ministry of Health. In addition, it provides support services for programme implementation by way of in-service training, provision of supplies and equipment for family health programmes and technical guidance.

Even though the indicators on maternal health are relatively satisfactory at the national level, it is necessary to pay attention to 'within country' variations, with several districts reporting high values[11].

Special groups

The inter-district variations in the MMR within Sri Lanka could be attributed, to a large extent, to the presence of selected population

Table 2 Key health-related indicators—Sri Lanka

Indicator	Year	Data	Source
Life expectancy at birth	1996–2001		Department of Census
Total		73.0	and Statistics
Female		75.4	
Male		70.7	
Total fertility rate (per woman)	1995–2000	1.9	Demographic and Health Survey 2000
Maternal mortality rate (per 10,000 live births)	1996	2.3	Registrar General's Department
Pregnant women immunized with tetanus toxoid (%)	2001	88.7	Epidemiological Unit
Percentage of deliveries attended by trained personnel	2000	96	Demographic and Health Survey 2000
Percentage of live births in government hospitals	2001	92.0	Medical Statistics Unit
Women of childbearing age using contraceptives (%)	2000		Demographic and Health Survey 2000
Modern methods		49.5	
Traditional methods		20.5	
Per capita health expenditure (Rs)	2001	1.6	Department of Health Services
Public Health Midwives (per 100,000 population)	2001	24.9	Medical Statistics Unit
Hospital beds per 1000 population	2001	3.1	Medical Statistics Unit

Source: Annual Health Bulletin 2001, Ministry of Health, Sri Lanka.

groups, the two main groups being those in the plantation sector and those affected by the ongoing conflict situation.

Plantation sector

The plantations of Sri Lanka date back to the colonial times when South Indian labour was brought to work in the labour intensive tea plantations. The health of the immigrant worker was the responsibility of the plantation management. The unsatisfactory health status of the immigrant labour led to the enactment of the Medical Wants Ordinance No. 17 of 1875. This specified the provisions to be made by the employer towards meeting the obligation to provide medical care. There were no special provisions for MCH services under this Ordinance. Provision of MCH services should have been a high priority as a major component of the work force included women of child-bearing age.

In the 1930s, the services were provided through a system of dispensaries and a few hospitals, in charge of estate dispensers and apothecaries. In the 1940s, some persons residing on the estates were trained as midwives. There were no major changes in the provision of MCH services in the estates, until the acquisition of estates by the government, under the Land Reform Law, in 1974/75. In 1974, the Family Health Bureau of the Ministry of Health commenced on an estate MC service.

The development of maternal health services was similar to those in the non-estate health services. Trained midwives, family welfare supervisors, Assistant Medical Practitioners and Estate Medical Assistants provided the services. Women were provided with transport facilities and paid leave to attend antenatal clinics.

With changing economic policies and the restructuring of the plantation industry, the management of the plantations was gradually transferred to the private sector, so that by 1998, with the exception of a few estates managed by the state sector, all others were managed by the private sector, which led to a complete change in the management of health and welfare services[21]. In the mid-1990s, the MMR was in the range of 0.9–1.9 per 1000 live births, higher than the reported figure for Sri Lanka. The difficult terrain and the long distances that these mothers had to travel to government institutions that provide emergency obstetric care may have contributed to some of these deaths. The future plans for the provision of maternal health services (a component of the total package of health care) seem to be uncertain, with some commitments being made by the state for providing such services.

Conflict-affected areas

The existence of a conflict situation in the northern and eastern part of Sri Lanka dates back nearly two decades. The districts of the north and east were the areas that were most involved in the conflict and the areas adjoining these districts were also affected to some extent. Assessment of the current status of the health services indicates the need for targeted programmes especially for the displaced populations, disruption of health services to varying degrees, non-availability of personnel and inadequate data on population and health status[22].

Limited data indicate a higher maternal mortality ratio and a high proportion of home deliveries (19.4% for the North East and 41% for Batticaloa district) along with a higher total fertility rate of 2.6 (Sri Lanka 1.9), all indicating that developing appropriate strategies is an urgent need.

Challenges for the future

With much emphasis placed on health sector reforms in recent years and the constraints faced by the state sector for provision of health care, maintaining the coverage and quality of maternal health services is indeed a challenge.

In the current scenario, where the MMR is relatively low, improving the quality of data not only for maternal mortality but also for morbidity is a priority. It is necessary to consider improving the current system of maternal death audit by establishing a system for confidential inquiry into maternal deaths.

Information available in recent years indicates the increasing importance of 'indirect causes' of maternal deaths, indicating the need for innovative strategies to minimize such events.

Maternal morbidity is still an area that has not received adequate attention in the MCH services in Sri Lanka, even though some initiative has been made in this regard, in recent years. Though there is a widespread network of institutions in Sri Lanka, equity in geographical access to emergency obstetric care still needs to be considered[23]. Another challenge will be to develop appropriate programmes to reduce inter-district variations in MMR with special reference to the plantation sector and the conflict-affected areas.

Acknowledgement

We wish to thank Dr Madura Wickrama for assistance in collating data.

References

1 *Population by Sex, Age, Religion, Ethnicity According to District and D.S. Division, 2001.* Census of Population and Housing 2001. Ministry of Finance and Planning, Department of Census and Statistics Census of Population and Housing, 2001

2 *Economic and Social Statistics of Sri Lanka 2002.* Colombo, Sri Lanka: Central Bank of Sri Lanka, 2002

3 *Annual Health Bulletin 2000.* Colombo, Sri Lanka: Ministry of Health, 2001

4 Uragoda CG. *A History of Medicine in Sri Lanka.* Colombo, Sri Lanka: Sri Lanka Medical Association, 1987

5 *Administration Report of the Director of Medical and Sanitary Services, 1948.* Ceylon: Department of Medical and Sanitary Services, 1949

6 *Administrative Report of the Director of Health Services, 1967.* Colombo, Ceylon: Department of Health Services, 1968

7 *Administrative Report of the Director of Health Services, 1954.* Colombo, Ceylon: Department of Health Services, 1955

8 *Administrative Report of the Director of Health Services, 1955.* Colombo, Ceylon: Department of Health Services, 1956

9 *Administration Report of the Director of Medical and Sanitary Services, 1947.* Ceylon: Department of Medical and Sanitary Services, 1949

10 *Administration Report of the Director of Medical and Sanitary Services, 1947.* Ceylon: Department of Medical and Sanitary Services, 1948

11 *Annual Health Bulletin 2001.* Colombo, Sri Lanka: Ministry of Health, 2002

12 *Administration Report of the Director of Medical and Sanitary Services, 1948.* Ceylon: Department of Medical and Sanitary Services, 1949

13 Pathmanathan I, Lilijestrand J, Martins JM, Rajapakse LC, Lissner C, de Silva A, Selvaraju S, Singh PJ. *Investing in Maternal Health.* Washington, DC: The World Bank, 2003; 105–50

14 *Sri Lanka Demographic and Health Survey 1987.* Ministry of Plan Implementation, 1989

15 *Sri Lanka Demographic and Health Survey 1993.* Department of Census and Statistics Ministry of Finance, Planning, Ethnic Affairs and National Integration in collaboration with the Ministry of Health, Highways and Social Services, 1995

16 *Sri Lanka Demographic and Health Survey 2000.* Department of Census and Statistics in collaboration with the Ministry of Health, Nutrition and Welfare, 2002

17 *Annual Health Bulletin 1993.* Colombo, Sri Lanka: Ministry of Health, 1994

18 Bandutilleka THC. *Epidemiology of Maternal Mortality on Sri Lanka.* MD Thesis. Colombo: Postgraduate Institute of Medicine, 1996

19 *Annual Report of Family Health.* Colombo, Sri Lanka: Evaluation Unit, Family Health Bureau, Ministry of Health, 2000

20 Gunatilleka G. Sri Lanka's social achievements and challenges in social development and public policy. In: Daram Ghar (ed) *Social Development and Public Policy: A Study of Some Successful Experiences.* London: Macmillan, 2000

21 Vidyasagara NW. Health care in the plantation sector. *J Commun Physicians Sri Lanka Millennium Suppl* 2001; 29–41

22 *Health System and the Health Needs of the Northeast Sri Lanka.* Colombo, Sri Lanka: World Health Organization, 2002

23 *Needs Assessment Study. Women's Rights to Life and Health Project.* Colombo, Sri Lanka: Ministry of Health, 2001

Unsafe abortion: the silent scourge

David A Grimes

Department of Obstetrics and Gynecology, University of North Carolina School of Medicine, Chapel Hill, North Carolina, USA

An estimated 19 million unsafe abortions occur worldwide each year, resulting in the deaths of about 70,000 women. Legalization of abortion is a necessary but insufficient step toward improving women's health. Without skilled providers, adequate facilities and easy access, the promise of safe, legal abortion will remain unfulfilled, as in India and Zambia. Both suction curettage and pharmacological abortion are safe methods in early pregnancy; sharp curettage is inferior and should be abandoned. For later abortions, either dilation and evacuation or labour induction are appropriate. Hysterotomy should not be used. Timely and appropriate management of complications can reduce morbidity and prevent mortality. Treatment delays are dangerous, regardless of their origin. Misoprostol may reduce the risks of unsafe abortion by providing a safer alternative to traditional clandestine abortion methods. While the debate over abortion will continue, the public health record is settled: safe, legal, accessible abortion improves health.

Introduction

*Correspondence to:
Dr D A Grimes,
Department of Obstetrics
and Gynecology,
CB# 7570, University of
North Carolina School of
Medicine, Chapel Hill,
NC 27599-7570, USA.
E-mail: dagrimes@
mindspring.com*

The tragedy of unsafe abortion goes largely unnoticed, a silent scourge in developing countries. Were a jumbo jet carrying 400 women of reproductive age to crash today in Central Africa, with loss of all lives on board, the response would be prompt and predictable. International press coverage would start within hours, with television crews and teams of investigators pouring over the smoking wreckage in search of the cause. Reporters would dutifully interview grieving relatives. Imagine the global response if yet another identical jet, loaded to capacity with women younger than 45 years, met the same fate a few days later in Southeast Asia. Then another in South America. And another in the Caribbean. Suppose that, over a year, 168 such airliners went down, killing all on board. How long would governments of the world allow such an airplane to fly before demanding corrective action?

Burden of suffering

Year in and year out, this many women (about 70,000) die of complications of unsafe abortion[1]. An estimated 19 million desperate women each year risk degradation, disease and death through such abortions[2]. The response of the international community remains muted, perhaps in part because the victims are all women, they are mostly of colour, and they live in developing countries. They die in places like Ouagadougou, not Oslo. Their deaths are all the more tragic, since nearly all are preventable.

More is known today about the epidemiology of legally induced abortion than any other operation. In contrast, huge gaps persist in our understanding of the incidence, morbidity and mortality of unsafe abortion. Because of stigma[3] or fear of legal reprisals, unsafe abortions are grossly under-reported, and the complications thereafter are often concealed or attributed to spontaneous miscarriage. For example, a recent hospital study from Ethiopia reported that 86% of abortions were spontaneous, yet the mean gestation age at admission was 15 weeks, an improbable scenario[4].

Despite gross under-reporting (due in part to deaths outside of hospital), unsafe abortion remains one of the five leading causes of maternal death in most developing countries[5-9]. For every woman who dies, many more are left wounded, some with life-long consequences, including infertility, chronic pelvic pain and genital trauma.

Through the leadership of the World Health Organization, several important publications in recent years have addressed the complex issue of unsafe abortion and its remedies. These include review articles[1,10], books[11] and the May 2002 issue of *Reproductive Health Matters*. Since the social and political approaches to the problem of unsafe abortion have been explored in detail in these references, I will focus on the medical aspects. This article will review the scope of the problem and address strategies for prevention and treatment of unsafe abortion and its sequelae.

Definition

'Unsafe abortion' is defined by the World Health Organization as 'a procedure for terminating an unwanted pregnancy either by persons lacking the necessary skills or in an environment lacking the minimal medical standards or both'[2]. Of note, 'unsafe' is not a synonym for 'illegal' or 'clandestine'. For example, legal abortions may be unsafe because of poorly trained clinicians, inadequate facilities, or both.

Potential solutions

Legalization of abortion

Legalization of abortion can dramatically improve women's health. Several natural experiments reveal the potential. In the USA, for example, the legalization of abortion led to the emptying and then closing of septic abortion wards in major metropolitan hospitals[12]. On a nationwide basis, deaths from illegal abortion nearly disappeared within a few years of nationwide legalization[13].

The opposite was observed in Romania after abortion was made inaccessible by the dictator Ceaucescu. Birth rates remained stable, but maternal mortality rates soared to the highest in Europe. Women resorted to unsafe abortion to control their fertility, and many died. When Ceaucescu was deposed and abortion again became accessible, maternal mortality rates plummeted[14].

More recently, Poland severely restricted abortion after decades of easy access. The result has been an estimated 80,000–200,000 clandestine abortions annually, women travelling to other countries for service, an increase in the cost of abortion, and no change in birth rate[15]. Clearly, the public health has suffered as a result.

Legalization of abortion, although important, is insufficient. India has had legal abortion on the books for several decades, as has Zambia. However, the 'devil is in the details'. In both countries, numerous impediments to care, ranging from requirement for several doctors' signatures to lack of accessible clinics, prevent most women in need from getting care in a timely fashion[10]. Hence, women continue to rely on unsafe abortion to control their fertility.

A companion article in this issue recounts the South African experience. A recent analysis of the public health impact of legalization of abortion in 1997 found little benefit. However, the low uptake (abortion ratio 36 per 1000 live births; abortion rate 3 per 1000 women aged 12–49 years)[16] suggests a large unmet need for safe, legal abortion. By comparison, the corresponding abortion ratio and rate for the USA are 264 and 17, respectively[17]. Hence, many women in South Africa probably still resort to unsafe practices[18].

Improving access

Removing needless barriers to abortion is fundamentally important. In the USA, for example, the response of general hospitals to the nationwide legalization of abortion in 1973 was tantamount to default; even today, most do not provide abortions. Out of this service vacuum arose free-standing abortion clinics, which now provide most abortions in the USA. They offer greater convenience, lower costs and greater safety than do hospitals[19].

Women in developing countries often must run a gauntlet to get a safe abortion. Problems include the metropolitan concentration of abortion providers, consent to contraceptive sterilization as a prerequisite, lack of an appointment system and hefty charges for services that should be free[10]. Lack of confidentiality of providers regarding minors poses another obstacle for adolescents. Even in India, where abortion has been legal for three decades, most women in one survey were unaware that it was legal[20].

Improving clinical care

Abortion providers vary widely in both quantity and quality. Even where abortion is legal, providers may be limited in both number and in skill. Many clinicians have little training for induced abortion. Experience with spontaneous abortion, where the cervix is often dilated, is not analogous to induced abortion. Many clinicians continue to use obsolete instruments, such as the metal curette. Moreover, limited evidence suggests that mid-level clinicians, such as physician's assistants and midwives, are competent to provide not only care of complications[21] but also to perform first-trimester abortions themselves[22].

Upgrading facilities

Simple, inexpensive equipment is needed for providing abortion services and caring for most complications that occur. Elaborate operating theatre set-ups and availability of general anaesthesia, required by some bureaucracies as a prerequisite for licensing[20], are inappropriate. Provided that arrangements and transportation (*e.g.* a jeep-taxi in rural India or a speedboat in Bangladesh) are in place for quickly moving patients to hospitals, if needed, free-standing abortion clinics around the world have achieved an outstanding safety record. Although abortion equipment is simple, it must be available. A major barrier to care in many developing countries is the lack of basic equipment and drugs for all gynaecological care[23].

Legal abortion in the first trimester: lessons learned

Determinants of safety

Two principal determinants of the safety of legally induced abortion are gestational age and choice of method. Both are closely interrelated. Abortion morbidity as a function of gestational age plots as a 'J'-shaped curve. The nadir for complication rates by vacuum aspiration occurs at 7–10 weeks from last menses. Among first-trimester surgical procedures, suction curettage is superior to sharp curettage in speed, comfort and safety. The metal curette, introduced in 1843 by Recamier to 'scrape off uterine fungosities'[24], sparked an immediate, strident debate. Scanzoni protested that the metal curette was 'an instrument based on an entirely erroneous thought, which takes from it all practical utility'. A century and a half later, solid evidence supports Scanzoni's dim view of the metal curette; it should be relegated to museums.

Anaesthesia

Local anaesthesia is safer than general anaesthesia for early abortion; it is cheaper as well. Indeed, in some countries, general anaesthesia is the leading cause of death from early abortion. However, local anaesthesia is not without risks. Toxicity and occasional deaths can occur if clinicians exceed safe doses of local anaesthetic agents, especially those of the amide class (lignocaine family). In the USA, no deaths have been attributed to local anaesthesia with ester anaesthetics (procaine family), although their use is less common. In general, clinicians should use the smallest amount of the lowest concentration adequate for the purpose. For example, 1% lignocaine is one of the more toxic local anaesthetic agents; using a 0.5% solution provides excellent anaesthesia with a wider margin of safety.

Cervical priming

Cervical preparation for surgical abortion can facilitate the operation. Osmotic dilators, such as naturally occurring laminaria or synthetic devices made of polyvinyl alcohol sponge impregnated with magnesium sulphate or hygroscopic plastic, have been used selectively. In recent years, misoprostol has gained wide use for this purpose. A dose of 400 µg given vaginally 2–3 h before the planned operation provides dilation that is often adequate to perform early suction curettage[25]. Should subsequent dilation be required, tapered dilators of the Pratt or Denniston design require much less force than do Hegar dilators[26]. Hegar dilators, like metal curettes, are antiques from the 19th century.

Tissue inspection

Formal pathology examination of the uterine contents is unnecessary. In contrast, visual inspection of the aspirate by the clinician or a designee is mandatory before the patient leaves the facility. A number of women have died from unsuspected ectopic pregnancies in this setting. Confirmation of the appropriate type and volume of tissue excludes ectopic pregnancy (except for the rare ectopic twin) as well as failed attempted abortion. The requisite equipment is simple: a source of back-lighting (such as a horizontal X-ray viewing box), a mesh kitchen strainer and a shallow transparent dish (like that used for baking pies). When the rinsed tissue is suspended in water and examined with back-lighting, this simple set-up allows immediate identification of embryonic tissue as early as 5 weeks and recognition of molar pregnancy as well.

Pharmacological approaches

Pharmacological abortion has transformed the landscape over the past decade. In recent years, the term for drug-induced abortion in early pregnancy has been 'medical' abortion. This ambiguous term has caused needless confusion and thus needs to be replaced with a more descriptive term. For example, in many cultures, 'medical' abortion implies that performed by medical personnel, such as physicians or midwives. Thus, in some countries, a vacuum aspiration performed by a physician would be deemed a 'medical' abortion, as compared with an abortion induced by a lay person.

Several approaches to pharmacological abortion are used, depending on the local availability of drugs. The best appears to be the combination of mifepristone followed by misoprostol. A popular regimen includes an oral dose of mifepristone 200 mg by mouth followed 1–3 days later with vaginal misoprostol, up to 800 μg. The optimal regimen has not been established, and research is under way to evaluate different doses and routes of administration (*e.g.* buccal or sublingual misoprostol). Regimens of mifepristone and misoprostol have been found safe and effective in both developed and developing countries[27].

Where mifepristone is not available, another alternative is methotrexate 50 mg/m^2 as a single intramuscular injection, followed some days later by misoprostol. This rivals the success of mifepristone–misoprostol, although the process is slower. Although many clinicians use blood tests to ensure normal liver function before administering single-dose methotrexate, the necessity of this practice is unclear. Another option more widely available is misoprostol alone. Reports suggest that the success of this approach is not as high as with the combined drug regimens, and gastrointestinal toxicity and fever become problems with repetitive doses[28].

Ancillary measures

Several ancillary measures lower morbidity as well. All patients having vacuum aspiration abortions should receive prophylactic antibiotics, although the optimal regimen remains unclear[29]. Doxycycline is popular, given its low cost, high safety and wide spectrum. Rh-negative women should receive Rh immunoglobulin.

Midtrimester legal abortion: lessons learned

Surgical abortion

Second-trimester abortion can also be performed surgically or pharmacologically. Through about 16 weeks, dilation and evacuation (D&E) is superior to labour-induction abortions. The comparative safety and acceptability of D&E *versus* labour-induction abortion at later gestational ages are currently unknown. Studies with abortifacients no longer used, such as intra-amniotic $PGF_{2\alpha}$, showed that D&E was superior to labour induction. One recent cohort study from a US hospital showed D&E to be significantly safer than labour-induction abortion, but selection bias was evident[30]. Randomized controlled trials comparing contemporary regimens with D&E are needed to resolve this question. D&E has several appealing features for developing countries, including reducing reliance upon scarce hospital beds and resources[31].

Pharmacological abortion

Several pharmacological approaches are used for labour induction. Intra-amniotic instillation of hypertonic saline (200 cc of 20%) or urea (80 g) remain safe and effective regimens. Augmentation by oxytocin, prostaglandin and osmotic cervical dilators shortens abortion times greatly. An advantage of hypertonic abortifacients is the lower risk of an abortus with signs of life; a disadvantage is a small risk of coagulopathy.

Uterotonic agents alone are effective abortifacients. One alternative is high-dose intravenous oxytocin, given in increasing concentrations[32]. This avoids the gastrointestinal distress associated with prostaglandins but requires many vials of oxytocin, which may be prohibitively expensive in developing countries. With scheduled breaks in the oxytocin infusion, water intoxication is avoided. Misoprostol alone, given by different routes and in different doses, can be effective as well[33]. An advantage is the low cost and wide availability of misoprostol; a disadvantage is dose-related gastrointestinal side-effects and fever. In countries where available, mifepristone administered before uterotonic agents dramatically reduces induction-to-abortion times.

Unsafe abortion

Choice of methods

The range of abortion methods used varies widely in safety and efficacy. Oral abortifacients have included quinine, ampicillin, laundry bluing, turpentine, bleach, acid, tea made of livestock faeces and other vegetable concoctions. Potassium permanganate tablets and herbal preparations have been used vaginally. Foreign bodies inserted through the cervix include sticks, roots, wires, knitting needles, coat hangers, rubber catheters and bougies, ball-point pens, bicycle spokes and chicken bones[34]. The last foreign body has led to unexplained infertility[35]. Physical methods have included abdominal massage[36], and lifting of heavy weights.

In the past, more invasive methods, *e.g.* introducing foreign bodies into the uterus, were more effective in producing abortions. They also tended to carry greater risks of trauma and infection. In one study from the Ivory Coast, plant infusions carried a high risk of neurotoxicity and maternal death, while intrauterine approaches were related to peritonitis[37].

Access to misoprostol has changed the landscape of unsafe abortion in several ways. First, it provides safe entrée into medical care. In many countries where legal abortion is not available, women induce vaginal bleeding by inserting a foreign body through the cervix. Once a diagnosis of 'spontaneous' incomplete or inevitable abortion is made, the woman can have a uterine aspiration with appropriate medical care. Misoprostol can cause such bleeding without the risk of instrumentation. In one report from Brazil, the infection rate associated with misoprostol was significantly lower than that with alternative traditional methods[38]. Second, if given in sufficient doses and with sufficient frequency, misoprostol alone can abort a high proportion of pregnancies.

Types of providers

A broad array of personnel perform unsafe abortions. Aside from the woman herself, others include physicians working at clandestine sites or in hospital operating theatres after hours. Others with medical experience include midwives, traditional birth attendants, pharmacists and nurses. Most worrisome are 'untrained quacks' whose motives may be financial and their skills negligible[39,40].

Ancillary measures

While the benefit of prophylactic antibiotics for vacuum aspiration has been established, the advisability of prophylaxis after other types of abortion is unclear. A recent Cochrane review has found the evidence too sparse to reach a conclusion[41]. Rh immune globulin should be given as indicated.

Treatment of complications

Incomplete abortion

The treatment of incomplete abortion is uterine evacuation. For decades, the assumption was that surgical removal was necessary. For first-trimester spontaneous abortion, that tenet has been challenged. Watchful waiting (expectant management) may be preferable, both in terms of emotional and physical welfare[42].

Alternatively, oxytocin has been used for decades to help expel tissue. More recently, misoprostol has attracted great attention as a uterotonic agent in this setting. A randomized controlled trial comparing surgical evacuation *versus* pharmacological evacuation with misoprostol found the latter to have fewer immediate complications; however, about half of those randomized to receive misoprostol later required surgical treatment. A Cochrane review in progress will compare expectant management with surgical intervention of miscarriage; another will compare medical (pharmacological) management of miscarriage.

Should surgical intervention be elected, suction curettage is preferable to sharp curettage[41]. Vacuum aspiration (suction curettage) with either an electrical pump or syringe as vacuum source is the standard of practice. For management of incomplete second-trimester abortion, pharmacological agents or surgical evacuation are options. Specially designed grasping forceps for D&E procedures, such as the Bierer or Sopher forceps, can quickly empty a large uterus, whereas labour-induction methods may take hours. Time can be critical when severe infection or heavy bleeding occurs. Hysterotomy to produce abortion (or to manage abortion) is an obsolete operation. This approach is needlessly risky, painful and expensive. Alternative means of emptying the uterus are preferable.

Haemorrhage

While oxytocic agents can assist, the definitive treatment of haemorrhage usually is to empty the uterus. Should uterine trauma or coagulopathy be responsible, specific treatment is indicated. More commonly, however, the task is to remove remaining tissue and help the uterus contract. Massage of the uterus, or firm, sustained compression between a vaginal and abdominal hand, can help temporize.

Should surgical evacuation be necessary, this should not be delayed to allow for correction of anaemia. Young, healthy women tolerate operations with very low haematocrits. Prompt resuscitation with volume expanders, rather than red cells, and rapid transfer to the operating theatre are appropriate. Although colloids, such as albumin, dextran 70, hydroxyethyl starches and plasma protein fraction, have been widely recommended for fluid resuscitation, a Cochrane review found them of comparable benefit to crystalloids, which are much less expensive. Hence, the latter should be used[43].

Infection

As with most gynaecological infections, the microbiology of post-abortal infection reflects the resident flora in the lower genital tract. Hence, antibiotic coverage should include Gram-positive organisms, Gram-negative rods and anaerobes. Some women will have involvement with sexually transmitted pathogens. When foreign bodies are involved, *Clostridium perfringens* needs to be considered as well.

Antibiotic coverage will depend on local availability, but two-drug therapy should be considered for serious infections. Examples include those mentioned by the Centers for Disease Control and Prevention for treatment of pelvic inflammatory disease, such as cefotetan plus doxy-cycline, or gentamicin plus clindamycin. Parenteral therapy is preferred, although if gut function is adequate, doxycycline can be administered orally with excellent serum levels obtained. Should the patient not respond appropriately, the possibilities of retained tissue, perforation, abscess formation and bowel injury need to be considered and evaluated.

A common practice in some developing countries is to allow several days of antibiotic therapy (sometimes only oral tetracycline) for clinical improvement before removal of retained tissue. Based on considerable indirect evidence[37,40,44], this delay appears dangerous. Serum levels of antibiotics will be achieved within an hour, and if the patient has stable vital signs, she should undergo evacuation promptly. The mainstay of treatment is emptying the uterus, and antibiotics will not succeed until the necrotic, infected tissue is removed. The common theme in fatal septic abortion is delay: delay in recognition, delay in getting to care, then delay in initiating care upon arrival.

Septic shock

Septic shock remains an important cause of death from unsafe abortion. The cornerstones of management include treatment of infection and cardiovascular support. For example, adult respiratory distress syndrome develops in one-quarter to one-half of such patients, and this complica-tion itself carries a high risk of death. High-dose, broad-spectrum antibiotics are indicated; no evidence indicates that triple antibiotics are preferable to two drugs.

Recently published systematic reviews have examined several ancillary treatments of sepsis and septic shock. Corticosteroids appear worthless and, indeed, may be harmful. They should not be used[45]. Naloxone[46] and intravenous polyclonal immunoglobulin[47] appear promising, but more research is needed. Drotrecogin alpha also improves survival in severe sepsis, but is expensive[48].

Should the patient not respond, laparotomy is advisable. Similarly, abdominal exploration is usually indicated for uterine perforation with suspicion of organ injury, clostridial myometritis with intramural gas formation and suspected or confirmed pelvic abscess.

Bowel trauma

Bowel injury is a common consequence of uterine perforation, either with pointed instruments or grasping forceps. The distal ileum appears to be most vulnerable to injury, followed by the sigmoid[49]. Figure 1 depicts small

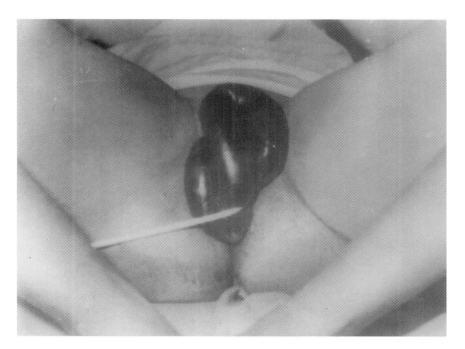

Fig. 1 Loops of gangrenous small intestine protruding from the vagina, 20-year-old patient at 16 weeks' gestation, Lagos University Teaching Hospital, Lagos, Nigeria. Reproduced from Oye-Adeniran BA, Umoh AV, Nnatu SSN. Complications of unsafe abortion: a case study and the need for abortion law reform in Nigeria. Reproduced from *Reprod Health Matters* 2002; **10**: 18–21 with permission from Elsevier.

bowel herniated through a perforation of the utero-vesical space during an attempted midtrimester abortion; the uterus was intact. Resection and reanastomosis of the necrotic bowel were required to save the patient's life.

Injuries of the colon are easier to recognize than are small-bowel injuries, because of prompt peritoneal soiling. A normal or declining white blood count can be deceiving—a harbinger of septic shock. In general, any woman with abdominal pain after uterine instrumentation should be considered to have a perforation with bowel injury until proven otherwise. In the face of faecal contamination and severe peritonitis, colorectal injuries should not be repaired primarily. Diverting colostomy with take-down some months later is prudent. Patients should be advised about and consented for colostomy whenever a laparotomy is performed in this setting. As with other contaminated cases, the wound should have a delayed primary closure.

'Too little, too late'

Lack of training, unfamiliarity with treatment options, out-of-stock drugs, broken equipment, sporadic electricity and water, and transportation challenges all threaten the health of women grappling with unsafe abortion[23]. Perhaps the greatest danger of all is indifference—or overt disdain.

The lack of commitment on the part of medical and nursing staff to provide prompt, attentive and emotionally supportive care indirectly dooms women whose lives could easily be saved. Many women who reach medical facilities are met with suspicion and hostility, and their treatment deferred while other more 'suitable' candidates receive medical attention[10]. When dealing with patients in need, judgemental behaviour on the part of health care personnel is both medically dangerous and ethically indefensible.

While the debate over the role of abortion in society will continue unabated, the public health record is clear[13]. Safe, legal and accessible abortion improves the health of women and their families. When medical historians look back upon our era, the legalization of abortion will stand out, along with the development of antibiotics and immunization, as a public health triumph.

Table 1 Suggested websites on abortion

http://gynpages.com/	Abortion clinics on-line
http://www.acog.com/	American College of Obstetricians and Gynecologists
http://www.cdc.gov/	Centers for Disease Control and Prevention
http://www.crlp.org	Center for Reproductive Law and Policy
http://www.guttmacher.org/	Alan Guttmacher Institute
http://www.ipas.org/	Ipas
http://www.popcouncil.org/	The Population Council
http://www.prochoice.org/	National Abortion Federation
http://www.rcog.org.uk/	Royal College of Obstetricians and Gynaecologists
http://www.who.int/en/	World Health Organization

Table 2 Key points for clinical practice

- Legalization of abortion is temporally associated with profound improvements in women's health, and vice versa
- Vacuum aspiration or pharmacologic methods are safe and effective for early abortion
- Sharp curettage is obsolete and should be abandoned
- Misoprostol given before vacuum aspiration primes the cervix for operation
- Prophylactic antibiotics should be given to all women having vacuum aspiration; evidence is insufficient concerning miscarriage and unsafe abortion patients
- Delays in treating complications of unsafe abortion further compromise safety
- Crystalloids are preferable to colloids for volume expansion
- Corticosteroids are worthless in septic shock; drotrecogin alpha improves survival
- Any woman with abdominal pain after an abortion should be considered to have a uterine perforation with bowel injury until proven otherwise

References

1 Van Look PF, Cottingham JC. Unsafe abortion: an avoidable tragedy. *Best Pract Res Clin Obstet Gynaecol* 2002; **16**: 205–20

2 Ahman E, Shah I. Unsafe abortion: worldwide estimates for 2000. *Reprod Health Matters* 2002; **10**: 13–7

3 Johnson-Hanks J. The lesser shame: abortion among educated women in southern Cameroon. *Soc Sci Med* 2002; **55**: 1337–49

4 Yusuf L, Zein ZA. Abortion at Gondar College Hospital, Ethiopia. *East Afr Med J* 2001; **78**: 265–8

5 Ganatra B, Johnston HB. Reducing abortion-related mortality in South Asia: a review of constraints and a road map for change. *J Am Med Womens Assoc* 2002; **57**: 159–64

6 Olatunji AO, Sule-Odu AO. Maternal mortality at Sagamu, Nigeria—A ten year review (1988–1997). *Niger Postgrad Med J* 2001; **8**: 12–5

7 Verma K, Thomas A, Sharma A, Dhar A, Bhambri V. Maternal mortality in rural India: a hospital based, 10 year retrospective analysis. *J Obstet Gynaecol Res* 2001; **27**: 183–7

8 Granja AC, Machungo F, Gomes A, Bergstrom S. Adolescent maternal mortality in Mozambique. *J Adolesc Health* 2001; **28**: 303–6

9 Fawole AA, Aboyeji AP. Complications from unsafe abortion: presentations at Ilorin, Nigeria. *Niger J Med* 2002; **11**: 77–80

10 Berer M. Making abortions safe: a matter of good public health policy and practice. *Bull World Health Organ* 2000; **78**: 580–92

11 Mundigo AI, Indriso C. *Abortion in the Developing World*. New Delhi: Vistaar Publications, 1999

12 Seward PN, Ballard CA, Ulene AL. The effect of legal abortion on the rate of septic abortion at a large county hospital. *Am J Obstet Gynecol* 1973; **115**: 335–8

13 Cates W Jr. Legal abortion: the public health record. *Science* 1982; **215**: 1586–90

14 Abortion: one Romania is enough. *Lancet* 1995; **345**: 137–8

15 Girard F, Nowicka W. Clear and compelling evidence: the Polish tribunal on abortion rights. *Reprod Health Matters* 2002; **10**: 22–30

16 Jewkes R, Brown H, Dickson-Tetteh K, Levin J, Rees H. Prevalence of morbidity associated with abortion before and after legalisation in South Africa. *BMJ* 2002; **324**: 1252–3

17 Herndon J, Strauss LT, Whitehead S, Parker WY, Bartlett L, Zane S. Abortion surveillance— United States, 1998. *MMWR Surveill Summ* 2002; **51**: 1–32

18 Rutgers S. Two years maternal mortality in Matebeleland north Province, Zimbabwe. *Cent Afr J Med* 2001; **47**: 39–43

19 Grimes DA, Cates W Jr, Tyler CW Jr. Comparative risk of death from legally induced abortion in hospitals and nonhospital facilities. *Obstet Gynecol* 1978; **51**: 323–6

20 Iyengar K, Iyengar SD. Elective abortion as a primary health service in rural India: experience with manual vacuum aspiration. *Reprod Health Matters* 2002; **10**: 54–63

21 Miller S, Billings DL, Clifford B. Midwives and postabortion care: experiences, opinions, and attitudes among participants at the 25th Triennial Congress of the International Confederation of Midwives. *J Midwifery Womens Health* 2002; **47**: 247–55

22 Freedman MA, Jillson DA, Coffin RR, Novick LF. Comparison of complication rates in first trimester abortions performed by physician assistants and physicians. *Am J Public Health* 1986; **76**: 550–4

23 Rogo KO, Aloo-Obunga C, Ombaka C *et al.* Maternal mortality in Kenya: the state of health facilities in a rural district. *East Afr Med J* 2001; **78**: 468–72

24 Grimes DA. Diagnostic dilation and curettage: a reappraisal. *Am J Obstet Gynecol* 1982; **142**: 1–6

25 Singh K, Fong YF, Prasad RN, Dong F. Vaginal misoprostol for pre-abortion cervical priming: is there an optimal evacuation time interval? *Br J Obstet Gynaecol* 1999; **106**: 266–9

26 Hulka JF, Lefler HT Jr, Anglone A, Lachenbruch PA. A new electronic force monitor to measure factors influencing cervical dilation for vacuum curettage. *Am J Obstet Gynecol* 1974; **120**: 166–73

27 Winikoff B, Sivin I, Coyaji KJ *et al.* Safety, efficacy, and acceptability of medical abortion in China, Cuba, and India: a comparative trial of mifepristone–misoprostol versus surgical abortion. *Am J Obstet Gynecol* 1997; **176**: 431–7

28 Creinin MD, Pymar HC. Medical abortion alternatives to mifepristone. *J Am Med Womens Assoc* 2000; **55**: 127–32, 150

29 Sawaya GF, Grady D, Kerlikowske K, Grimes DA. Antibiotics at the time of induced abortion: the case for universal prophylaxis based on a meta-analysis. *Obstet Gynecol* 1996; **87**: 884–90

30 Autry AM, Hayes EC, Jacobson GF, Kirby RS. A comparison of medical induction and dilation and evacuation for second-trimester abortion. *Am J Obstet Gynecol* 2002; **187**: 393–7

31 Cates W Jr, Schulz KF, Grimes DA. Dilatation and evacuation for induced abortion in developing countries: advantages and disadvantages. *Stud Fam Plann* 1980; **11**: 128–33

32 Owen J, Hauth JC, Winkler CL, Gray SE. Midtrimester pregnancy termination: a randomized trial of prostaglandin E2 versus concentrated oxytocin. *Am J Obstet Gynecol* 1992; **167**: 1112–6

33 Jain JK, Kuo J, Mishell DR Jr. A comparison of two dosing regimens of intravaginal misoprostol for second-trimester pregnancy termination. *Obstet Gynecol* 1999; **93**: 571–5

34 Polgar S, Fried ES. The bad old days: clandestine abortions among the poor in New York City before liberalization of the abortion law. *Fam Plann Perspect* 1976; **8**: 125–7

35 Hunger C, Ring A. [Chicken bones in the uterus—an exceptional reason for sterility]. *Zentralbl Gynakol* 2001; **123**: 604–6

36 Sambhi JS. Abortion by massage—'bomoh'. *IPPF Med Bull* 1977; **11**: 3

37 Goyaux N, Yace-Soumah F, Welffens-Ekra C, Thonneau P. Abortion complications in Abidjan (Ivory Coast). *Contraception* 1999; **60**: 107–9

38 Faundes A, Santos LC, Carvalho M, Gras C. Post-abortion complications after interruption of pregnancy with misoprostol. *Adv Contracept* 1996; **12**: 1–9

39 Rogo KO. Induced abortion in sub-Saharan Africa. *East Afr Med J* 1993; **70**: 386–95

40 Thapa PJ, Thapa S, Shrestha N. A hospital-based study of abortion in Nepal. *Stud Fam Plann* 1992; **23**: 311–8

41 May W, Gulmezoglu AM, Ba-Thike K. Antibiotics for incomplete abortion. *Cochrane Database Syst Rev* 2000; CD001779

42 Nielsen S, Hahlin M. Expectant management of first-trimester spontaneous abortion. *Lancet* 1995; **345**: 84–6

43 Alderson P, Schierhout G, Roberts I, Bunn F. Colloids versus crystalloids for fluid resuscitation in critically ill patients. *Cochrane Database Syst Rev* 2000; CD000567

44 Grimes DA, Cates W Jr, Selik RM. Fatal septic abortion in the United States, 1975–1977. *Obstet Gynecol* 1981; **57**: 739–44

45 Cronin L, Cook DJ, Carlet J *et al.* Corticosteroid treatment for sepsis: a critical appraisal and meta-analysis of the literature. *Crit Care Med* 1995; **23**: 1430–9

46 Boeuf B, Gauvin F, Guerguerian AM, Farrell CA, Lacroix J, Jenicek M. Therapy of shock with naloxone: a meta-analysis. *Crit Care Med* 1998; **26**: 1910–6

47 Alejandria MM, Lansang MA, Dans LF, Mantaring JB. Intravenous immunoglobulin for treating sepsis and septic shock. *Cochrane Database Syst Rev* 2002; CD001090

48 Bernard GR, Vincent JL, Laterre PF *et al.* Efficacy and safety of recombinant human activated protein C for severe sepsis. *N Engl J Med* 2001; **344**: 699–709

49 Imoedemhe DA, Ezimokhai M, Okpere EE, Aboh IF. Intestinal injuries following induced abortion. *Int J Gynaecol Obstet* 1984; **22**: 303–6

Abortion: developments and impact in South Africa

RE Mhlanga

Department of Health, Pretoria, Republic of South Africa

The article seeks to clarify the context of the Choice on Termination of Pregnancy Act, 1996 (Act No.92 of 1996), the factors that led to its adoption and implementation including the role of research in support of policy development, the expanded utilization of professional nurses, and the respect and promotion of women's right to life and well-being. The challenges that cropped up on the road to implementation and sustenance are also spelt out. It is important to evaluate the programme because this will assist South Africa to improve on the performance of service delivery. It will also assist other countries, both poor and rich, to progressively realize the promotion of human rights. Lastly, the article also seeks to identify areas that will lead to the improvement of women's lives, and ultimately societal development and health.

Introduction

South Africa reformed the abortion law in order to improve the health of women and prevent deaths among women. It is arguably one of the most significant steps in respecting the rights of women to choice and to bodily integrity. The Act—the Choice on Termination of Pregnancy Act, 1996—represents a departure from the past where the woman was always regarded as a minor irrespective of her age or marital status. It also represents a departure from the philosophy that the doctor would always know what is best, and make a decision based on his or her judgment. Access to safe pregnancy termination is easier, and maternal deaths from illegal abortions, though still occurring are reduced. The challenges to access include information availability, rurality, attitude of health workers and communities, and limited resources for counselling. The stigma attached to termination of pregnancy is something that the health system and health care community has to deal with.

Correspondence to:
Dr RE Mhlanga, Cluster
Manager, Maternal, Child
and Women's Health and
Nutrition, Department of
Health, Pretoria, Republic
of South Africa. E-mail:
mhlane@health.gov.za

British Medical Bulletin 2003; 67: 115–126
DOI: 10.1093/bmb/ldg006

Background

South Africa has a high maternal mortality rate, especially among the African population. Septic abortion is a major contributor to maternal death incidence rates. Various studies had shown the incidence, extent and terrible consequences of unsafe abortion. However, little could be done because of the prevailing legal environment at that time. Under the Hippocratic Oath, abortion upon request or demand is prohibited. During the time before the passing of the Abortion and Sterilization Act, 1975 (Act No.2 of 1975), the application of the prohibition of abortion was so severe that one eminent gynaecologist and obstetrician was struck off the medical register. Hardly 3 years later, the Sterilization and Abortion Act, 1975 was passed and enacted in record time. This practitioner has had to live with the stigma and the consequences of that ruling.

The history of women is intimately linked to the history of the oppressed, in that women were not allowed to make any decision with regard to their lives, including their reproductive lives. Because of the continued morbidity and mortality among women of all races, the National Party government of South Africa introduced a law in the 1970s, the Abortion and Sterilisation Act, 1975 (Act No.2 of 1975). That Act sought to make abortion accessible under certain circumstances. The conditions that had to be fulfilled were so stringent that only women in urban and well-resourced areas could make use of the provisions of the Act. Many women who would benefit from the Act stayed in rural areas where only one or two doctors were present in a hospital, and therefore abortion could not be permitted, as the law required that at least three doctors agree that the woman needed a legal abortion! Some women from richer families or who could afford went overseas to procure termination of pregnancy. The Act therefore was part of the response to the need to protect the lives of the privileged (mostly white population), while neglecting the welfare of the many women who were in the rural areas, and who did not know of the facilities that could be available for legal abortion. Even the presence of such knowledge would hardly help as provincial hospitals were governed by the apartheid laws that forbade Blacks from utilizing White hospitals. This led to women seeking help in the unhealthy environments of backstreet rooms. The majority of these women died or suffered severe morbidity.

Women are responsible for caring for the family, yet they are marginalized when it comes to employment. They are oppressed because of their lack of access to financial resources. This then makes them vulnerable to be abused, for the sake of having a sure source of income. Men often take advantage of this compromised position. Women also depend on men to provide finances for them to access health care, with the result that women tend to present late for medical attention. In developing countries, poverty has a woman's face.

South Africa is a strongly Calvinistic country, with other religions such as Roman Catholicism and Islam having a substantial affiliation. The apartheid Government influenced the church practices, and it was influenced by the church in its policies. The church also provided theological justification for the policies of South Africa. There is now a growing charismatic religious movement within the country, with varying levels of conservative persuasions with regard to reproductive and family health.

With the political liberation of South Africa in 1994, it was imperative that laws should start responding to the needs of the majority, and women were among those who needed their human rights respected, protected and promoted. South Africa started responding to the reproductive health needs of women by tackling one of the most contentious issues—abortion. South Africa was responding to the recommendations of the International Conference on Population and Development (ICPD) and the United Nations Convention on the Elimination of All Forms of Discrimination against Women (CEDAW).

The religious sector was engaged, though not comprehensively, but since the Act has been passed, there are continuing consultations and workshops to involve all sectors, especially men, in the promotion of reproductive health and contraception. The traditional leaders are also engaged in discussions so that they support this initiative. Community mobilization using acceptable messengers is very important.

After much debate and support from research institutions and academic institutions showing the burden of ill-health and death from septic abortion, and the need for legislative reform, the South African government passed the Choice on Termination of Pregnancy Act, 1996 (Act No.92 of 1996). Health workers provided inputs on the likely positive impact of easier access to safe termination of pregnancy services. The Act has a preamble, stressing that it would and should not be used as a method of contraception. Its passage was concomitant to strengthening contraception services and providing alternatives to women who would not be desirous or able to bring up children from unwanted pregnancies.

Contents of the Act

Among the prerequisites to termination of pregnancy is the requirement that information must be provided with regard to alternatives that are available to the woman with regard to the unwanted pregnancy. The alternatives include foster parenting, adoption and maintenance.

The Act also allows registered midwives to undergo training in termination of pregnancy, and to provide the service for women who are up to 12 weeks pregnant (by dates).

A year later, the Ministry of Health established the National Committee for the Confidential Enquiry into Maternal Deaths (NCCEMD), and made maternal deaths notifiable. The NCCEMD investigates all maternal deaths notified, and makes recommendations to the Minister every 3 years. The committee makes special recommendations with regard to the termination of pregnancy (TOP) services in the country. This then places the Choice on Termination of Pregnancy Act, 1996 squarely in the strategy for reducing maternal mortality and morbidity.

The Act broadened conditions under which a pregnancy can be terminated. It divides the gestational period into three parts for the sake of termination of pregnancy.

1   Up to and including 12 weeks gestation by dates.

2   Above 12 weeks up to and including 20 weeks gestation by dates.

3   Above 20 weeks gestation by dates.

The Act allows doctors and midwives who are skilled to terminate a pregnancy up to and including 12 weeks gestation. Only doctors are allowed to terminate pregnancies above 12 weeks under certain conditions. The Act has thus reduced the upper limit from the 28 weeks that is traditionally accepted as the cut-off point for viability. The Act also governs the termination of pregnancy up to and including viability, thus including induction of labour and caesarean section.

A woman of any age may request termination of her pregnancy without having to advance reasons for such, on condition the pregnancy is not more than 12 weeks gestation. After 12 weeks gestation, termination of pregnancy can only be carried out under certain conditions. These are: pregnancy having been the result of rape, severe fetal abnormality, severe maternal physical or mental disease, or if continued pregnancy would result in severe social or economic conditions. A pregnancy over 12 weeks but not more than 20 weeks may only be terminated upon the recommendation of a midwife or a medical practitioner, and upon the consent of the woman. It is of note here that the consent of the spouse, guardian or parent(s) is not required.

One of the features of the Act is the respect for women's right to choose, irrespective of the age of the woman who is pregnant. The Act requires that health workers advise a child to consult with a parent, guardian or a family friend before the termination of a pregnancy. However, if the child chooses not to inform anyone, access to termination of pregnancy services shall not be denied her. The clause was deemed necessary given that there are children who may have been sexually abused by their guardians or parents. If the permission of the parents or guardian were necessary, it would pose a barrier to seeking help. It is this part which also poses difficulties in some circles.

The Act also makes provision for counselling before termination of pregnancy, though this is optional. Elements of information that must be made available to the woman include alternate options to the pregnancy termination. These include foster parenting, child support grant, adoption and maintenance from the biological father of the unborn child. The Act makes it possible for women who are considered minors to access termination of pregnancy without the consent of the parent(s) or guardian.

Regulations were developed and these set out criteria for facilities wishing to offer surgical termination of pregnancy. These regulations also established norms and standards for performing the procedure. The safety of the woman is the prime concern of the Act, and anyone terminating a pregnancy must be competent to do so, and must have easy and ready access to supportive equipment and resuscitation facilities. There must also be ready access to emergency transport should this become necessary.

In summary, therefore, the Act sets the limit of 20 weeks gestation as the boundary for viability, considering the first day of the last normal menstrual period. All pregnancies above 20 weeks gestation are considered in the same light as any viable pregnancy. The termination of such a pregnancy must be in accordance with normal midwifery and obstetric practice. Therefore, there are fewer grounds for termination of pregnancy as the pregnancy progresses. It is also based on the woman requesting termination of her pregnancy. It provides for the minimum information that must accompany the service. The Act allows midwives to carry out termination of pregnancy if they have the skills to do so. The Act also makes it an offence for anyone other than a trained health worker to provide pregnancy termination services. Facilities have to fulfil certain set criteria in order to qualify for termination of pregnancy.

Clinical challenges

Though the Choice on Termination of Pregnancy Act was passed in 1996, it was only implemented in 1997, as the health system had to prepare and train health workers. A dilemma arose when women would present for termination of pregnancy before its enactment. The other challenge involved health workers who objected to participate in termination of pregnancy service provision. The Constitution of the Republic of South Africa protects the rights of workers not to participate on grounds of religion or personal conviction. This continues to be a challenge.

The challenges to implementing the Act lay in the provision of access to safe practices. The sudden freedom to choose would result in many women wanting to access the service. The approach was to obtain equipment [manual vacuum aspiration (MVA) in this case], drugs and people to perform the pregnancy termination. There was also the real danger that radical elements within the so-called Pro-Life movement would target health care providers. The challenge lay, therefore, in getting opposing factions to work together for the lives of women and children.

Women became frustrated by delays and deliberate obstruction to pregnancy termination services. Women would then access misoprostol to initiate the abortion, and present at health facilities with vaginal bleeding. Objecting (to the Act) hospital doctors and nurses would then refuse to attend to these women. The Health Professions Council of South Africa had to remind doctors that their duty was to attend to the woman who is bleeding.

The health services have difficulty in providing second trimester abortions. This is because many women at this gestational age require admission, and the Act allows only doctors to perform the procedure.

One of the provinces took the decision to centralize the TOP facilities within one major hospital until enough health workers were trained to decentralize the service. All the other hospitals would refer the women (or couples) to the hospital and bear the responsibility of providing transport for the women. This has worked very well, and access to TOP services has improved steadily over the years. The service has now largely been decentralized to district level in this province.

Training

In South Africa, as in many other countries, gynaecological procedures are performed by trained doctors only. Doctors are trained to perform termination of pregnancy as part of their competencies during the internship year. However, it was necessary to equip nurses to perform the pregnancy termination, as there are very few doctors in the underserved areas, especially the rural areas. The demand for the service would also increase, thus overwhelming the available resources.

The methods for termination of pregnancy consisted of surgical evacuation of the pregnant uterus. The limitation of this became obvious early in the process, as the need for anaesthesia would make termination of pregnancy inaccessible where there are no skilled doctors to administer this. The MVA technique became the method of choice. However, few doctors in South Africa were familiar with the MVA of the products of conception. Dilatation of the cervix depended on either very expensive drugs such as prostaglandin tablets or gel.

Experiences elsewhere had shown the usefulness of misoprostol as a cervical ripening agent, as well as an abortifacient if used in conjunction with mefipristone. British experiences and practice informed the use of misoprostol. However, the company that made misoprostol would not consent to including pregnancy termination as an added indication for the use of the drug. The medical profession in South Africa has continued to use this drug for cervical ripening, as comparable drugs are unaffordable.

During the early phase of consultations before the Bill was put before parliament, there was consideration of the use of medical abortion. The requirements that France had put in indicated that there must be strict oversight for the completion of pregnancy termination. Such oversight could not be assured within the South African public health sector. Many women who would otherwise benefit from this would not be able to return for review to ensure that evacuation of the pregnant uterus has been complete. The alternative would be to admit the women until they have aborted. This is also not sustainable because of limited space within facilities. The issue of off-label use of misoprostol also became significant. For this reason, medical termination of pregnancy could not be entertained as a public health programme.

The training would therefore aim at providing TOP services at the lowest level of the health system as possible. Training involved the following:

- Values clarification workshops

- Identification of adequate numbers of midwives and doctors for the provision of TOP care

- Training in MVA for both doctors and nurses

- Development of management guidelines, including the use of prostaglandin analogues, especially misoprostol

- Contraception including emergency contraception, as pregnancy termination had to be accompanied by contraception counselling and advice

The Department and partners for the promotion and protection of human rights supported the health care workers through visits and refresher courses. Non-governmental organizations assisted in training for counselling and for provision of TOP services.

Research

It became necessary to monitor and evaluate the quality of TOP services from the beginning. The opposition required evidence, and the benefits of the service had to outweigh the disadvantages. It was also necessary to look at newer and easier ways for conducting abortions so that the service could be provided at primary health care level. An advisory group of practitioners was constituted to carry out these functions. They looked at, among other things, the appropriate route for administration and the recommended dosage of misoprostol. The group also looks into ways of improving service delivery. It is important that quality of service is an important component of monitoring progress.

Legal challenges

Soon after the implementation of the Act, a group of Christian professionals challenged the Act in a court of law. The group alleged that the Choice on Termination of Pregnancy Act, 1996 was unconstitutional based on right to life. The contention was that a fetus, irrespective of gestational age, has a claim to protection by the Constitution for its right to life, because it is a person. While the State recognizes the progressive development towards personhood, the fetus is not a person in law until its first breath at birth. Support for the pro-life lobby action came from, among others, the USA. The court, however, found in the State's favour.

Another court case against the State was initiated recently by the same organization. As mentioned before, the Act has not found favour with all and sundry, particularly some of the religious organizations. The particular organization is objecting to the right of persons under the age of 18 years to having the right to make a decision on the future of their pregnancy without the consent of their parents. The point of view of the Department of Health is that the woman, once pregnant, should be in a state to make decisions about her own health and that of the fetus. The age of the woman is then of secondary importance. With the increase in reported sexual abuse, sometimes by a close relative, it means that some of the unwanted pregnancies are the result of rape by close relatives or friends of the family. It also means that the woman (adult or child) will be under extreme pressure not to report to the police or to terminate a pregnancy.

Impact

Since the implementation of the Act in 1997, there has been a dramatic increase in the number of pregnancy terminations in public health care institutions. The private sector has also responded to the need to provide the services.

The maternal mortality, though insensitive to immediate changes, if disaggregated yields important information. The process of maternal

Table 1 Incidence (%) of severely ill women admitted with incomplete abortion

	1994	2000	*P*-value
Signs of infection			
None	79.5	90.1	0.0051
Offensive discharge	13.5	6.4	0.0041
Tender uterus	8.4	3.7	0.0794
Localized peritonitis	1.7	0.7	0.1863
Mechanical or chemical	3.2	0.6	0.002
Foreign body	1.3	0	0.00347
Management of incomplete abortion			
Antibiotics given	43.6	33.5	0.2384
Blood/blood products	13.4	8.3	0.1
Sharp curettage	97.6	82	0.0045
N	803	761	

There was a reduction in the percentage of women who presented ill and required intensive management. Although the total numbers of women with incomplete abortions are the same, the reduction in the severely ill points to less pressure on women to keep the termination of their pregnancies.

The study was commissioned by the Department of Health in South Africa to study the impact of the Choice on Termination of Pregnancy Act, 1996. The study was carried out by the Reproductive Health Research Unit and the Medical Research Council that carried out the initial research before the passing of the new Act.

mortality therefore shows the changes that have occurred through the legal reform. There is a definite improvement in maternal deaths following septic abortion.

A recent study commissioned by the Department of Health showed that there is a decrease in the incidence of severely ill women admitted with incomplete abortion (Table 1). There was therefore less morbidity accompanying wilful and spontaneous abortion. The total number of women presenting with abortion, though, has not decreased significantly. This is explained in part by the fact that many women seek help at general practitioners' rooms. Because these facilities are not designated in terms of the Act, doctors then advise the women to present to a health facility as soon as they start bleeding after taking misoprostol. In this way, women present early when the process of abortion is already established, before sepsis can set in.

The Choice in Termination of Pregnancy has been accompanied by the use of misoprostol as a prostaglandin analogue. This has been a facilitating occurrence. However, this also has increased the illegal use of misoprostol by untrained people in order to induce abortions or labour. The incidence of the use of this and similar drugs is known, and the prevalence of unaborted fetuses that progress to term is not known.

Some health workers, especially some doctors, would refuse to attend to women bleeding if they suspected or knew that the pregnancy was terminated wilfully. The Health Professions Council of South Africa, the statutory body for medical practitioners, has issued a directive that any doctor refusing to treat a woman who is bleeding will be guilty of misconduct. The South African Nursing Council has also made a similar ruling.

The approach of the Choice on Termination of Pregnancy Act, 1996 is in line with the Human Rights Approach. Women's rights are human rights. The previous Act (Abortion and Sterilization Act, 1975) afforded access to safe termination of pregnancy for a select section of the population, and it benefited mostly urban and more affluent and white persons requiring assistance with an unwanted pregnancy.

Because of the religiosity of the country, many people are opposed to the Choice on Termination of Pregnancy. The atmosphere under which health workers operate to implement this Act is therefore not supportive or enabling. The health workers are stigmatized and they need psychological support as well.

The Choice on Termination of Pregnancy Act, 1996 also opened the abortion issue for dialogue and debate. Radio, television, magazines and newspapers often carry space for debate on this topic. The heated and often malignant debates of the past are not witnessed that much these days, except under special circumstances in parliament.

Training of midwives

Many pregnancy terminations have been carried out by midwives who have been trained in the procedure of manual vacuum evacuation. These health workers are now so good that they are even better placed to teach medical practitioners in the safe termination of pregnancy procedures. The Act has been cautious in allowing registered midwives to perform termination of pregnancy. The rationale for this was consideration of the skills that registered midwives already have with regard to pregnancy and the changes associated with such a physiological state. However, on review of the performance of registered midwives during the first 5 years of implementing the Act, the South African Society of Gynaecologists and Obstetricians recommended that consideration be given to training other categories of registered nurses to perform pregnancy termination up to 12 weeks gestation.

It is critical to have guidelines with regard to diagnosis and management of pregnancy. Because of limited resources, emphasis is placed on history and clinical examination for determining uterine size (gestational age). A uterine size of 16 weeks, even with a confirmed fetal size of

10 weeks (by ultrasound), would not be appropriate for a nurse to manage, because of the increased chances of complications. A pregnancy in a scarred uterus is also not amenable for management by a nurse. Use of prostaglandins in these conditions requires skills and vigilance.

Termination of pregnancy is associated with stigma in many communities. This also applies to the working environment, where some doctors and nurses discriminate against those providing termination of pregnancy services. This has led to some nurses leaving the service after only a few months of TOP service provision.

In an environment where there is violence against women, and many pregnancies are unwanted, access to termination of pregnancy has provided an alternative to women who are desperate and are not in a position to bring up a child. The Act has laid the framework for the promotion and protection of the rights of women, and to the promotion of reproductive choices. With proper skills transfer and support, it is also evident that health workers other than medical doctors can provide safe termination of pregnancy.

The ultimate aim of the Choice on Termination of Pregnancy Act, 1996 is to prevent morbidity from unwanted pregnancy, and to make TOP services available and accessible to all women, especially those in rural areas.

Parliament has established a process through which it monitors the implementation of the Choice on Termination of Pregnancy Act, 1996. It has already held two public hearings in order to hear the voices of women and stakeholders. The Act is currently being reviewed with the intention of making facilities more accessible, and to broaden the category of health workers to be trained to provide abortion services.

Research on medical and surgical termination of pregnancy is continuing.

Conclusion

The success of this implementation also shows that it is possible for countries with limited resources to provide safer termination of pregnancy services, in a quest to reduce the number of maternal deaths from unwanted pregnancies and unsafe abortion practices. It is therefore important for the political leadership to make the environment supportive of women's right to make decisions with regard to their reproductive future. Making abortion safer should be part of a greater commitment and initiative to improve women's health.

Maternal mortality is still a major contributor to people's development in developing countries. Unsafe abortion is a major contributor to maternal death and maternal ill-health. The attitude of patriarchal societies makes abortion a taboo, and therefore abortion never becomes a topic in the agenda of many countries, despite its negative impact on the health of women and children. It may indeed be time for the medical community to review the Hippocratic Oath, and remove those parts that, among others, discriminate against women.

Ensuring women's rights is a political responsibility, and it is necessary for the political leadership to take the bold step, which is a necessary and human step, and commit the country to respecting, protecting and promoting women's rights. South Africa took the decision based on sound scientific reason to respect these rights. The challenge is to further entrench these rights, and to ensure that the people most in need of relief are accorded access to services to prevent unwanted pregnancies and to safely terminate pregnancy when the need arises. The scientific community must provide the necessary leadership and support for excellence in providing necessary services for those in need, especially those in greatest need in terms of equity.

The words of the former Minister of Health, Dr Dlamini-Zuma, during the debates on termination of pregnancy in 1995, are appropriate as a conclusion. 'No woman enjoys having a pregnancy terminated. Therefore as a society we should strive to prevent by caring. I shall be the happiest person, if, one day, even in the presence of the Choice on Termination of Pregnancy Act, no woman feels compelled to terminate her pregnancy!'

Mothers infected with HIV

James McIntyre

Perinatal HIV Research Unit, University of the Witwatersrand, Johannesburg, South Africa

The HIV/AIDS epidemic intersects with the problem of maternal mortality in many circumstances. The extent of the contribution of HIV/AIDS to maternal mortality is difficult to quantify, as the HIV status of pregnant women is not always known. HIV infection and AIDS-related deaths have become one of the major causes of maternal mortality in many resource-poor settings. HIV impacts on direct (obstetrical) causes of maternal mortality by an associated increase in pregnancy complications such as anaemia, post-partum haemorrhage and puerperal sepsis. HIV is also a major indirect cause of maternal mortality by an increased susceptibility to opportunistic infections such as *Pneumocystis carinii* pneumonia, tuberculosis and malaria. Appropriate antiretroviral therapy started in pregnancy could reverse the toll of HIV-related maternal mortality. Without such efforts and increased HIV prevention, the gains achieved by safe motherhood programmes will be lost in the future.

Two intersecting epidemics

Correspondence to:
Prof. James McIntyre,
Perinatal HIV Research
Unit, University of the
Witwatersrand, Chris Hani
Baragwanath Hospital,
PO Bertsham,
Johannesburg,
South Africa, 2013.
E-mail:
mcintyre@pixie.co.za

The HIV/AIDS epidemic intersects with the problem of maternal mortality in many circumstances. Almost half of the 42 million people living with HIV are women in their reproductive years[1]. Across the world, over 2 million HIV-infected women are pregnant each year, over 90% of them in developing countries, while close to 600,000 women die each year from complications of pregnancy and childbirth, the majority of them also in resource-constrained settings. The extent of the contribution of HIV/AIDS to maternal mortality is difficult to quantify, as the HIV status of pregnant women is not always known. Although programmes to prevent mother-to-child transmission of HIV have expanded dramatically in many countries over the past few years, most pregnant women in high prevalence areas still do not have access to HIV counselling and testing.

HIV infection rates in pregnant women range from below 1% to over 40% in different countries. The highest rates are still in Africa, although prevalence in some Asian countries has risen considerably. Prevalence rates have fallen in some areas, such as Uganda, and there are encouraging signs that rates in young women are beginning to fall in South Africa and some other sub-Saharan settings, but the prevalence remains high in

British Medical Bulletin, Vol. 67 © The British Council 2003; all rights reserved many others[1]. As the epidemic becomes more established in many countries, increasing numbers of pregnant women are being encountered who have been infected for longer and present with HIV/AIDS complications, which will impact on maternal mortality rates. By the mid 1990s in Tanzania, AIDS was the leading cause of death for women in the reproductive age group[2], a situation now common to many resource-poor countries. There is some evidence for a decrease in fertility in high HIV prevalence settings[3–5], which may reduce the risk of maternal mortality from AIDS-related causes, although HIV/AIDS remains the leading cause of death in adults in these areas[6].

HIV/AIDS may influence maternal mortality in several ways. Women living with HIV/AIDS may be more susceptible to direct or obstetric causes of maternal mortality, such as post-partum haemorrhage, puerperal sepsis and complications of caesarean section. AIDS-related deaths may be incidental to the pregnancy (fortuitous) or may be true indirect causes of maternal mortality where the infection itself or opportunistic infections such as tuberculosis progress faster in the pregnancy. There is growing evidence for the impact of the AIDS epidemic on maternal mortality rates and for the effect of AIDS-related complications on maternal deaths.

The effect of AIDS on maternal mortality: changing the causes of maternal mortality

The maternal mortality ratio (MMR) in resource-poor settings is 10–100 times that of industrialized countries. Rates in these countries can be over 1000 per 100,000 live births compared to less than 10 in resource-rich settings. In South Africa, where maternal mortality rates are lower than in most African countries, the MMR from the country's first national report on maternal deaths in 1998 was 12.3 times higher than that of the UK, partly attributable to HIV/AIDS[7]. In addition, severe maternal morbidity may be up to 10 times more common than mortality.

In the past, direct obstetric causes have been responsible for most of the deaths of mothers, with the majority attributed to haemorrhage, hypertension, obstructed labour and abortion complications. This pattern is changing in many places as AIDS-related complications now account for a high proportion of maternal deaths. The trio of AIDS, tuberculosis and malaria have become more important as causes of maternal mortality.

AIDS has also become a contributing cause of maternal mortality in developed countries, although much smaller in numbers, despite better access to appropriate care. Before the widespread availability of highly active antiretroviral therapy (HAART), AIDS was becoming a leading cause of maternal mortality in some areas of the USA. A retrospective study in New Jersey, USA, showed a rise in maternal mortality in the early 1980s, with a decrease in deaths from direct obstetric causes and AIDS the major cause of pregnancy-related mortality[8]. In areas of Europe with high levels of immigrant populations, a similar pattern is seen[9]. With better access to HAART, mortality has decreased in people with AIDS[10], and current treatment recommendations support the use of appropriate antiretroviral treatment in pregnant women[11,12], which will reduce the rates of AIDS complications seen during pregnancy. In most resource-poor settings, however, this level of treatment is unavailable to date, and HIV/AIDS remains a major problem[13].

Several African and Asian studies in the 1990s demonstrated the increasing role of AIDS and related illnesses as causes of maternal mortality. MMRs in these studies ranged from 400 to over 900 per 100,000 live births. A study in Zambia showed that rates of maternal mortality increased eight-fold over the past two decades, despite better obstetric services[14]. Indirect causes of maternal mortality were responsible for 58% of deaths, with malaria and AIDS-related tuberculosis the most common of these. In the Rakai district of Uganda, maternal mortality was five times higher in HIV-positive women than in HIV-negative women, reaching rates of over 1600 per 100,000 live births in the infected group[6]. In Malawi and Zimbabwe, pregnancy-related mortality has increased 1.9 and 2.5 times, in parallel with the increasing AIDS epidemic[15].

AIDS-related deaths were the primary cause of death in mothers in Brazzaville in 1993[16], while AIDS was the fourth highest cause of maternal mortality in a Tanzanian district[17]. In India, a study in AIDS symptomatic women showed high rates of maternal mortality. *Pneumocystis carinii* pneumonia (PCP) followed by miliary tuberculosis and wasting disease were the most common AIDS-defining illnesses and causes of maternal death[18].

In South Africa, a national confidential enquiry into maternal deaths was instituted in 1998. AIDS was the second most common cause of maternal death in 1998, accounting for 13% of all deaths in the first year[19]. In the years 1999–2001, AIDS was the listed cause of death in 17% of cases, although this figure may be considerably underestimated as HIV status was known in only 36% of cases[20].

Maternal dietary deficiencies may exacerbate the progression of HIV. Vitamin A deficiency has been shown to be associated with more rapid disease progression in HIV-infected women, increased rates of transmission of HIV from mother to child and higher levels of viral load in breast milk. Vitamin A supplementation has not been shown to reduce the risk of mother-to-child transmission, but there is little information on the effect on maternal health in HIV-infected women. A large study in a general population in Nepal showed that supplementation with vitamin A or beta carotene reduced maternal mortality by 44%[21]. In Tanzania, multivitamin supplementation, but not vitamin A alone, resulted in significant increases in CD4, CD3 and CD8 counts[22]. Further research may be indicated to investigate the role of vitamin supplementation in reducing maternal mortality and morbidity on HIV-positive women[23].

The effect of pregnancy on HIV/AIDS progression

Data available from developed countries suggest that pregnancy does not accelerate the progression of HIV disease[24–27]. A systematic review and meta-analysis of seven cohort studies from 1983 to 1996 suggested that there was an association between adverse maternal outcomes and pregnancy in HIV-infected women. The summary odds ratios for the risk of an adverse maternal outcome related to HIV infection and pregnancy were 1.8 (85% CI 0.99–3.3) for death, 1.41 (95% CI 0.85–2.33) for HIV disease progression and 1.63 (95% CI 1.00–2.67) for progression to an AIDS-defining illness. This association appeared to be stronger in the one study in this group conducted in a resource-poor setting.

The effect of HIV on mothers is not limited to the period included in maternal mortality figures, and figures correlating HIV infection and maternal mortality may underestimate the combined effects of the two conditions. While little effect on disease progression is described in the post-pregnancy period in resource-rich settings[28], or in Thailand[29], there is evidence from several studies in Africa that the mortality of HIV-infected women is also high in the post-pregnancy period.

In a prospective study of anti-malaria prophylaxis in over 4000 mothers in Malawi, the maternal mortality rate was 370 per 100,000 women and the mortality rate between 6 weeks and 1 year post-partum was 341 per 100,000 live births. AIDS and anaemia were the major causes of post-pregnancy mortality[30]. In Zaire, maternal mortality rates in HIV-infected women were 10 times those of HIV-negative women[31], with 22% of HIV-infected mothers dying during a 3-year follow-up period.

John and colleagues have shown an interesting correlation between CCR5 promoter polymorphisms and increased mortality post-pregnancy in a Kenyan cohort[32]. In this report, women with the 59356 C/T genotype had a 3.1-fold increased risk of death during the 2-year follow-up period (95% CI 1.0–9.5) and a significant increase in vaginal shedding of HIV-1-infected cells (odds ratio 2.1; 95% CI 1.0–4.3), compared with women with the 59356 C/C genotype. This suggests that there may be multiple factors, including nutritional and genetic, that influence the risk of faster progression during and post pregnancy.

Effect of HIV/AIDS on pregnancy complications

Obstetric causes of maternal morbidity and mortality may be more severe in women infected with HIV, and they may be more susceptible to infectious and post-surgical complications[25,33]. These include higher reported rates of ectopic pregnancy, early abortion, bacterial pneumonia, urinary tract infection, oral and recurrent vaginal thrush and other infections. Malaria and tuberculosis have become major complicating conditions in HIV-infected pregnant women. Anaemia may be much more frequent and severe in HIV-infected women, and especially so where pregnancy is complicated by malaria.

Post-partum and post-caesarean section complications have been described in some studies. Post-partum haemorrhage has been described as more common in some studies[17], and may be more serious if associated with pre-existing anaemia in HIV-infected women. Post-partum morbidity occurred in 15% of 1186 deliveries during 1990–1998 in The Women and Infants Transmission Study in the United States[34]. The most commonly reported post-partum morbidity events were: fever without infection, haemorrhage or severe anaemia, endometritis, urinary tract infection and caesarean wound complications. Post-caesarean section complications have been higher in some studies, particularly in those women who are severely immunosuppressed, but this is less likely where antibiotic prophylaxis is provided[35,36].

It has been suggested that the rate of pre-eclampsia is lower in HIV-infected women who do not receive antiretroviral treatment than in treated women or HIV-negative controls[37]. This association has not been confirmed to date in other cohorts. An underestimated cause of significant morbidity and some mortality in HIV-infected women is mental illness. A study in Zambia of women diagnosed as HIV-infected during pregnancy showed that the majority of women (85%) showed major depressive episodes and had significant suicidal thoughts[38].

HIV-related opportunistic infections

Several opportunistic infections associated with HIV infection may complicate pregnancy and cause maternal mortality. PCP has a more aggressive course during pregnancy, with an increase in both morbidity and mortality. Several case reports have illustrated the impact of PCP and the difficulties of treatment in pregnancy[39–42]. Other pulmonary diseases have been described more rarely in pregnancy, and these include bacterial infections (*Haemophilus influenzae* and *Streptococcus pneumoniae* along with *Pseudomonas aeruginosa*), fungal infections

(*Cryptococcus neoformans*, *Histoplasma capsulatum* and *Coccidioides immitus*), viral infections (cytomegalovirus) and opportunistic neoplasms (Kaposi's sarcoma, lymphoma)[43]. The extent to which pregnancy affects the course of these respiratory diseases in HIV-infected women is not well described. In general, management is similar to the non-pregnant state, but delays in diagnosis and treatment may influence the course of disease.

Less common but potentially fatal opportunistic infections described in pregnant women include disseminated herpes zoster[44] and cerebral toxoplasmosis[45].

Tuberculosis

One of the major contributing factors to maternal mortality in HIV-infected women is concurrent tuberculosis (TB) infection. TB is one of the leading infectious causes of death in women in the reproductive age group worldwide[46,47]. It is also the most common opportunistic infection associated with HIV in resource-poor settings, and the two epidemics of HIV and TB have had a synergic effect on each other.

An association between an increase in maternal mortality from TB was reported from Zambia in 1999[14]. A further study in Durban, South Africa, investigated 101 maternal deaths out of 50,518 deliveries[48]. In this group the MMR was 323 per 100,000 live births for HIV-infected mothers and 148 per 100,000 live births for HIV-negative mothers. The mortality rate for HIV and TB co-infection was 121/1000, three times that of TB without concurrent HIV infection. The authors concluded that 54% of maternal deaths due to TB were attributable to HIV infection. It is likely that this increased susceptibility to TB complications will continue to be a major cause of maternal mortality in high prevalence HIV areas[49,50].

Malaria

Over the past 5 years, there has been increasing evidence of an association between malaria in pregnancy and HIV infection[51–54]. HIV increases the risk of malaria in women of all gravidities, although the mechanism of this association is unclear. The standard recommended intermittent therapy regimens of sulfadoxine–pyrimethamine may be insufficient to clear parasitaemia in these women and may need to be reassessed[55].

Given the role of malaria as a potential cause of maternal mortality, the association of a higher prevalence of disease in HIV-infected women, the anaemia associated with both diseases and the potential interaction, more research is needed to determine appropriate control strategies.

Antiretroviral treatment

The major determinant of a fall in AIDS-related mortality in resource-rich settings has been the availability of antiretroviral treatment. In most resource-poor settings, antiretroviral treatment has not yet become widely available.

Guidelines from the United States Public Health Service, the World Health Organization and others recommend the appropriate use of antiretroviral treatment for pregnant women, as indicated by their clinical and immunological status[11,56].

If the impact of HIV on maternal mortality is to be controlled and reversed, appropriate use of antiretroviral treatment is essential[13]. While many countries have initiated programmes to reduce mother-to-child transmission of HIV, these will have to be expanded to include care of mothers. With increasing access to these drugs, health workers will have to be trained to identify women in need of treatment and to initiate and monitor treatment during pregnancy. Without such interventions, the efforts of safer motherhood and safe pregnancy programmes over the past two decades will be reversed as maternal mortality due to HIV/AIDS continues to rise.

References

1   UNAIDS/WHO. *AIDS Epidemic Update—December 2002*. UNAIDS/02.46E. Geneva: UNAIDS, 2002

2   Urassa E, Massawe S, Mgaya H, Lindmark G, Nystrom L. Female mortality in reproductive ages in Dar es Salaam, Tanzania. *East Afr Med J* 1994; **71**: 226–31

3   Zaba B, Gregson S. Measuring the impact of HIV on fertility in Africa. *AIDS* 1998; **12(Suppl. 1)**: S41–50

4   Gray RH, Wawer MJ, Serwadda D *et al*. Population-based study of fertility in women with HIV-1 infection in Uganda. *Lancet* 1998; **351**: 98–103

5   Hunter SC, Isingo R, Boerma JT, Urassa M, Mwaluko GM, Zaba B. The association between HIV and fertility in a cohort study in rural Tanzania. *J Biosoc Sci* 2003; **35**: 189–99

6   Sewankambo NK, Wawer MJ, Gray RH *et al*. Demographic impact of HIV infection in rural Rakai district, Uganda: results of a population-based cohort study. *AIDS* 1994; **8**: 1707–13

7   Mantel GD, Moodley J. Can a developed country's maternal mortality review be used as the 'gold standard' for a developing country? *Eur J Obstet Gynecol Reprod Biol* 2002; **100**: 189–95

8   Mertz KJ, Parker AL, Halpin GJ. Pregnancy-related mortality in New Jersey, 1975 to 1989. *Am J Public Health* 1992; **82**: 1085–8

9   Huss M, Bongain A, Bertrandy M, Hofman P, Grimaud D, Gillet JY. [Maternal mortality in Nice. Results of a reproductive age mortality survey using death registries in the Nice University Hospital, 1986–1993]. *J Gynecol Obstet Biol Reprod (Paris)* 1996; **25**: 636–44

10 Messeri P, Lee G, Abramson DM, Aidala A, Chiasson MA, Jessop DJ. Antiretroviral therapy and declining AIDS mortality in New York City. *Med Care* 2003; **41**: 512–21

11 Public Health Service Task Force. Recommendations for Use of Antiretroviral Drugs in Pregnant HIV-1-Infected Women for Maternal Health and Interventions to Reduce Perinatal HIV-1 Transmission in the United States. June 16, 2003

12   Connolly M, Nunn P. Women and tuberculosis. *World Health Stat Q* 1996; **49**: 115–9

13   Rosenfield A, Yanda K. AIDS treatment and maternal mortality in resource-poor countries. *J Am Med Womens Assoc* 2002; **57**: 167–8

14   Ahmed Y, Mwaba P, Chintu C, Grange JM, Ustianowski A, Zumla A. A study of maternal mortality at the University Teaching Hospital, Lusaka, Zambia: the emergence of tuberculosis as a major non-obstetric cause of maternal death. *Int J Tuberc Lung Dis* 1999; **3**: 675–80

15   Bicego G, Boerma JT, Ronsmans C. The effect of AIDS on maternal mortality in Malawi and Zimbabwe. *AIDS* 2002; **16**: 1078–81

16   Iloki LH, G'Bala Sapoulou MV, Kpekpede F, Ekoundzola JR. [Maternal mortality in Brazzaville (1993–1994)]. *J Gynecol Obstet Biol Reprod (Paris)* 1997; **26**: 163–8

17   MacLeod J, Rhode R. Retrospective follow-up of maternal deaths and their associated risk factors in a rural district of Tanzania. *Trop Med Int Health* 1998; **3**: 130–7

18   Kumar RM, Uduman SA, Khurrana AK. Impact of pregnancy on maternal AIDS. *J Reprod Med* 1997; **42**: 429–34

19   National Committee on Confidential Enquiries into Maternal Deaths. A review of maternal deaths in South Africa during 1998. National Committee on Confidential Enquiries into Maternal Deaths. *S Afr Med J* 2000; **90**: 367–73

20   National Committee on Confidential Enquiries into Maternal Deaths. *Saving Mothers 1999–2001*. Pretoria: Department of Health, South Africa, 2003

21   West Jr KP, Katz J, Khatry SK *et al*. Double blind, cluster randomised trial of low dose supplementation with vitamin A or beta carotene on mortality related to pregnancy in Nepal. The NNIPS-2 Study Group. *BMJ* 1999; **318**: 570–5

22   Fawzi WW, Msamanga GI, Spiegelman D *et al*. Randomised trial of effects of vitamin supplements on pregnancy outcomes and T cell counts in HIV-1-infected women in Tanzania. *Lancet* 1998; **351**: 1477–82

23   Tomkins A. Nutrition and maternal morbidity and mortality. *Br J Nutr* 2001; **85(Suppl. 2)**: S93–9

24   Bessinger R, Clark R, Kissinger P, Rice J, Coughlin S. Pregnancy is not associated with the progression of HIV disease in women attending an HIV outpatient program. *Am J Epidemiol* 1998; **147**: 434–40

25   McIntyre JA. *HIV in Pregnancy: A Review*. Occasional Paper No. 2. Geneva: World Health Organization, 1999

26   Weisser M, Rudin C, Battegay M, Pfluger D, Kully C, Egger M. Does pregnancy influence the course of HIV infection? Evidence from two large Swiss cohort studies. *J Acquir Immune Defic Syndr Hum Retrovirol* 1998; **17**: 404–10

27   Ahdieh L. Pregnancy and infection with human immunodeficiency virus. *Clin Obstet Gynecol* 2001; **44**: 154–66

28   Hocke C, Morlat P, Chene G, Dequae L, Dabis F. Prospective cohort study of the effect of pregnancy on the progression of human immunodeficiency virus infection. The Groupe d'Epidemiologie Clinique Du SIDA en Aquitaine. *Obstet Gynecol* 1995; **86**: 886–91

29   Manopaiboon C, Shaffer N, Clark L *et al*. Impact of HIV on families of HIV-infected women who have recently given birth, Bangkok, Thailand. *J Acquir Immune Defic Syndr Hum Retrovirol* 1998; **18**: 54–63

30   McDermott JM, Slutsker L, Steketee RW, Wirima JJ, Breman JG, Heymann DL. Prospective assessment of mortality among a cohort of pregnant women in rural Malawi. *Am J Trop Med Hyg* 1996; **55**: 66–70

31   Ryder RW, Nsuami M, Nsa W *et al*. Mortality in HIV-1-seropositive women, their spouses and their newly born children during 36 months of follow-up in Kinshasa, Zaire. *AIDS* 1994; **8**: 667–72

32   John GC, Bird T, Overbaugh J *et al*. CCR5 promoter polymorphisms in a Kenyan perinatal human immunodeficiency virus type 1 cohort: association with increased 2-year maternal mortality. *J Infect Dis* 2001; **184**: 89–92

33   Rodrigues J, Niederman MS. Pneumonia complicating pregnancy. *Clin Chest Med* 1992; **13**: 679–91

34   Read JS, Tuomala R, Kpamegan E *et al*. Mode of delivery and postpartum morbidity among HIV-infected women: the women and infants transmission study. *J Acquir Immune Defic Syndr* 2001; **26**: 236–45

35 Semprini AE, Castagna C, Ravizza M *et al.* The incidence of complications after caesarean section in 156 HIV-positive women. *AIDS* 1995; **9**: 913–7

36 Marcollet A, Goffinet F, Firtion G *et al.* Differences in postpartum morbidity in women who are infected with the human immunodeficiency virus after elective cesarean delivery, emergency cesarean delivery, or vaginal delivery. *Am J Obstet Gynecol* 2002; **186**: 784–9

37 Wimalasundera RC, Larbalestier N, Smith JH *et al.* Pre-eclampsia, antiretroviral therapy, and immune reconstitution. *Lancet* 2002; **360**: 1152–4

38 Kwalombota M. The effect of pregnancy in HIV-infected women. *AIDS Care* 2002; **14**: 431–3

39 Minkoff H, deRegt RH, Landesman S, Schwarz R. *Pneumocystis carinii* pneumonia associated with acquired immunodeficiency syndrome in pregnancy: a report of three maternal deaths. *Obstet Gynecol* 1986; **67**: 284–7

40 Ahmad H, Mehta NJ, Manikal VM *et al. Pneumocystis carinii* pneumonia in pregnancy. *Chest* 2001; **120**: 666–71

41 Albino JA, Shapiro JM. Respiratory failure in pregnancy due to *Pneumocystis carinii*: report of a successful outcome. *Obstet Gynecol* 1994; **83**: 823–4

42 Gates Jr HS, Barker CD. *Pneumocystis carinii* pneumonia in pregnancy. A case report. *J Reprod Med* 1993; **38**: 483–6

43 Saade GR. Human immunodeficiency virus (HIV)-related pulmonary complications in pregnancy. *Semin Perinatol* 1997; **21**: 336–50

44 Petrozza JC, Monga M, Oshiro BT, Graham JM, Blanco JD. Disseminated herpes zoster in a pregnant woman positive for human immunodeficiency virus. *Am J Perinatol* 1993; **10**: 463–4

45 O'Riordan SE, Farkas AG. Maternal death due to cerebral toxoplasmosis. *Br J Obstet Gynaecol* 1998; **105**: 565–6

46 Connolly M, Nunn P. Women and tuberculosis. *World Health Stat Q* 1996; **49**: 115–9

47 Diwan VK, Thorson A. Sex, gender, and tuberculosis. *Lancet* 1999; **353**: 1000–1

48 Khan M, Pillay T, Moodley JM, Connolly CA. Maternal mortality associated with tuberculosis–HIV-1 co-infection in Durban, South Africa. *AIDS* 2001; **15**: 1857–63

49 Pillay T, Khan M, Moodley J *et al.* The increasing burden of tuberculosis in pregnant women, newborns and infants under 6 months of age in Durban, KwaZulu-Natal. *S Afr Med J* 2001; **91**: 983–7

50 Corbett EL, Steketee RW, ter Kuile FO, Latif AS, Kamali A, Hayes RJ. HIV-1/AIDS and the control of other infectious diseases in Africa. *Lancet* 2002; **359**: 2177–87

51 Ladner J, Leroy V, Karita E, van de Perre P, Dabis F. Malaria, HIV and pregnancy. *AIDS* 2003; **17**: 275–6

52 Leroy V, Ladner J, Nyiraziraje M *et al.* Effect of HIV-1 infection on pregnancy outcome in women in Kigali, Rwanda, 1992–1994. Pregnancy and HIV Study Group. *AIDS* 1998; **12**: 643–50

53 van Eijk AM, Ayisi JG, ter Kuile FO *et al.* HIV increases the risk of malaria in women of all gravidities in Kisumu, Kenya. *AIDS* 2003; **17**: 595–603

54 Ayisi JG, van Eijk AM, ter Kuile FO *et al.* The effect of dual infection with HIV and malaria on pregnancy outcome in western Kenya. *AIDS* 2003; **17**: 585–94

55 Verhoeff FH, Brabin BJ, Hart CA, Chimsuku L, Kazembe P, Broadhead RL. Increased prevalence of malaria in HIV-infected pregnant women and its implications for malaria control. *Trop Med Int Health* 1999; **4**: 5–12

56 World Health Organization. *The Use of Essential Drugs: Eighth Report of the WHO Expert Committee (including the revised Model List of essential drugs). Technical Report Series No 882.* Geneva: World Health Organization, 1998

Malaria prevention strategies

M Cot and **P Deloron**

Institut de Recherche pour le Développement, UR 010, Paris, France

Acute and severe consequences of pregnancy-associated malaria (PAM), such as materno-fetal death or cerebral malaria, seem limited to unstable malaria areas. In areas of stable endemicity, the main consequences are maternal anaemia and low birth weight (LBW) babies, particularly in primigravidae. Placental malaria seems more frequent and its consequences more severe in HIV-infected women. Since 1964, several chemoprophylaxis controlled trials have been undertaken, mainly in Tropical Africa where malaria is stable. Most showed an increase in mean birth weight in the prophylaxis group, especially among primigravidae. Similar findings were made with anaemia. Prophylaxis seems less effective in the case of HIV–malaria co-infection, which may require an increase in the number of doses. At present, intermittent treatment with sulfadoxine–pyrimethamine given twice or thrice during pregnancy in antenatal clinics seems the best policy for preventing PAM. Such effective prophylaxis should be integrated with other antenatal clinic services. Recently identified molecular receptors involved in cytoadherence of parasitized erythrocytes to placenta could yield new therapeutic or vaccine approaches, specifically targeted to pregnant women.

Introduction

The burden of pregnancy-associated malaria in terms of perinatal death and morbidity is often mentioned but seldom incorporated into global initiatives that aim to improve the quality of health services for children and pregnant women, like Safe Motherhood (a partnership of national and international organizations, including UNICEF, WHO and the World Bank). The topic is generally studied by specialists of tropical disease rather than obstetricians or public health policy makers.

However, the impact of this disease during pregnancy was described nearly a century ago[1]. These early observations were undertaken during epidemics in areas of low transmission. They showed the particularly dramatic impact of malaria on the health of pregnant women as well as on the outcome of pregnancy. These first studies highlighted the high frequency of maternal deaths and high rates of abortions and stillbirths. Several investigations were subsequently undertaken in hyperendemic

Correspondence to:
Michel Cot, IRD UR 010,
Faculté de pharmacie,
Laboratoire de
parasitologie,
4 Avenue de
l'Observatoire,
75270, Paris Cedex 06,
France.
E-mail: Michel.Cot@ird.fr

areas, chiefly in the 1940s and the 1950s. These showed a lesser impact of malaria probably due to the acquisition of protective immunity by mothers living in these areas.

By the beginning of the 1980s, a general outline of the situation could be drawn[2], showing that the higher susceptibility of pregnant women to malaria and the association of low birth weight (LBW) and maternal anaemia to malarial infection of the placenta is a public health priority even in high transmission areas. At present, this problem is particularly important in sub-Saharan Africa, where it is estimated that, whereas 24 million women are exposed every year, fewer than 5% have access to effective interventions.

Consequences of malaria during pregnancy

Low endemicity areas

Ever since the first observations of epidemics, several epidemiological investigations have been carried out in different areas of low transmission[3-6]. The impact of unstable malaria on pregnant women varies according to the intensity of transmission. This is also true for the level of immunity acquired by mothers. The more severe complications of *Plasmodium falciparum* infection, such as cerebral malaria or pulmonary oedema (which can lead to maternal deaths), affect women with the lowest levels of immunity. Clinical malaria attacks with high fever and maternal anaemia are also frequent in areas of lower endemicity and affect primigravidae and multigravidae indifferently. Abortion, stillbirth and LBW are frequent consequences for the fetus (see Table 1).

Table 1 Clinical effects of pregnancy-associated malaria

		Stable malaria	Unstable malaria
Mother	Severe malaria (including death)	–	+
	Severe anaemia	+++ (mainly primigravidae)[a]	+++ (all parities)
	Hyperpyrexia	+	+++
	Placental infection	+++ (mainly primigravidae)[a]	+
Fetus/neonate	Abortion/stillbirth	–	++
	Symptomatic congenital Malaria	–	+
	LBW	+++ (mainly primigravidae)[a]	+++ (all parities)

+++: very common; ++: common; +: infrequent; –: rare.
[a]In the case of HIV co-infection, all parities seem to be affected.

High endemicity areas

In settings with stable transmission of *P. falciparum* malaria, over a hundred studies were published on pregnancy-associated malaria from 1950 to 1990, most involving large samples of women. Comprehensive reviews of these studies have been undertaken[2,7–9]. Their conclusions are generally in agreement, and very different from the observations made in areas of unstable malaria (see Table 1).

Maternal morbidity and mortality

Parasitaemia is more frequent and parasite density is higher during the first and, to a lesser extent, the second pregnancy, than in multigravidae or in non-pregnant women. Clinical signs of malaria are not frequent (*e.g.* fever).

Anaemia is more frequent in pregnant women, and more pronounced in primigravidae than in multigravidae[10–13]. The aetiology of anaemia in pregnancy is multifactorial. Causes such as poor nutrition (which induces iron and folate deficiencies), haemoglobinopathies and infection with other parasites (mainly hookworm) add to this syndrome. Most studies show a strong association between malarial infection of the placenta or peripheral blood and haemoglobin levels, confirming that this is a major cause of anaemia, even when other factors are present[12,13].

The effect of maternal anaemia on the course and the outcome of pregnancy is difficult to establish. If WHO standards are considered (haemoglobin < 11 g/dl), it appears that a very large proportion of pregnant women living in malaria-endemic areas should be considered anaemic [*e.g.* 72% in the Democratic Republic of Congo (former Zaire)[11] or 94% in Papua-New Guinea[14]]. Such mild anaemia does not seem to cause serious problems during pregnancy, as shown by recent studies conducted in developed countries[15] as well as in malaria-endemic countries[5,14]. In fact, only severe malaria (defined as haemoglobin < 7 g/dl or haemoglobin < 8 g/dl, depending on the authors[13,14,16]) can be associated with adverse perinatal outcomes, such as maternal mortality (by increasing the severity of postpartum haemorrhage) or LBW of the baby. Prevalence of severe anaemia (< 7 g/dl) in highly malaria-endemic zones varies greatly according to the study area (< 3% in the Democratic Republic of Congo[11], 9–10% in Tanzania and coastal Kenya[12,13]). There is a general lack of information on the outcomes for mothers and babies. However, in a comprehensive review of all studies published between 1985 and 2000, Steketee *et al*[9] estimated that maternal anaemia contributed to 7–18% of LBW and to 25% of total infant mortality.

Maternal mortality is difficult to estimate in tropical countries where there is a paucity of reliable data. This is particularly true of deaths related to malaria, which have been found to be associated with an increase in pre-eclampsia or postpartum haemorrhage. In addition to the difficulty of assessing a causal relationship between the two factors, the main problem is that diagnosis of malaria is usually based on either clinical examination or verbal autopsy, thus lacking specificity. Parasitological proof is not available in most cases. Based on a review of 23 studies in Africa, Brabin and Verhoeff[17] estimated that 0.5–23% of maternal deaths in hospital settings and 2.9–17.6% in community-based studies are due to malaria. It is interesting to note that one of the most reliable studies, set in Malawi in 1989, reported only 0.9% of deaths directly attributable to malaria. A year-long follow-up of 4053 pregnant women did not show an association between mortality and parasitaemia for mothers[18].

Placental malaria infection

Parasitaemia of the maternal placental blood is more frequent than parasitaemia of the maternal peripheral blood. This affects 10–34% of all pregnant women, depending on the studies[2,7,8], and primigravidae are more heavily and more often infected (up to twice as much) than multigravidae.

Fetal and newborn morbidity

All studies show a constant association between placental infection and LBW, which has a strong impact on neonatal and infant morbidity, particularly for first births. The mean decrease in birth weight associated with placental infection ranges from 55 to 348 g (all parities), equivalent to roughly a two-fold increase in the proportion of LBW, which usually affects 10–15% of births in malaria-endemic areas[2,6,7]. Although no complete understanding of the biological mechanism by which placental infection causes LBW has been reached, the combination of intrauterine growth retardation and prematurity is strongly suspected[7,14,19]. The overall contribution of maternal malaria to LBW is estimated to be 8–14% of all deliveries in malaria-endemic areas[9].

It is also difficult to assess the impact of maternal malaria infection on perinatal and infant mortality. Based on the few studies available, Steketee et al.[9] estimated that pregnancy-associated malaria was responsible for 3–8% of infant deaths (approximately 75,000–200,000 infants every year).

Transplacental infection of the newborn was established as of the 1930s, and its frequency varies highly according to published studies[20] (0–29%). No clear explanation has been found to understand such divergence in highly endemic areas. It seems that congenital infection of the baby is well tolerated in such settings, as no adverse effect was reported. Rapid parasite clearance in newborns was observed in the absence of antimalarial treatment in two studies[20,21].

HIV–malaria interaction

Since the onset and the rapid spread of the AIDS epidemic in areas where malaria transmission occurs, questions have arisen concerning a possible interaction between both infections. As HIV infection occurs in 3–27% of pregnant women in areas where malaria is present[9], this could represent a major public health problem. The first observations in Malawi, where nearly 3000 pregnant women were followed between 1987 and 1989, showed an increase in the parasite prevalence and density in HIV-positive compared with HIV-negative women[22]. These findings were recently confirmed by two studies in Malawi and Kenya[23,24]. Moreover, several studies[22,24] have noted that the usual pattern of increased parasite prevalence and density in primigravidae is altered. HIV-positive primigravidae are at similar risk of malaria as HIV-positive multigravidae.

There are indications that malaria can increase viral loads and mother-to-child HIV transmission[9,25], but this is largely an unresolved question.

Dual infection also influences the outcome of pregnancy. It seems that primigravidae with both infections have a two-fold increase in the risk of delivering a LBW baby compared with women infected with HIV alone[26].

Effect of malaria prevention strategies

Chemoprophylaxis

The first published randomized trial of chemoprophylaxis by pyrimethamine was carried out in Kenya in 1964[27]. It was followed by over 30 clinical trials comparing various drugs and regimens, more or less appropriate in terms of randomization and methodology. We refer here to systematic reviews that have been made of these studies[7,28,29].

Table 2 displays a list of the few drugs that are available for prophylaxis in pregnant women, along with their strengths and limitations. Table 3 is a selection of some of the main trials (prophylaxis *versus* placebo or no intervention) from 1964 to the present, showing a great variety of protocols, interventions, outcomes and results.

Regardless of their protocol, all published studies clearly show an important decrease in parasitaemia (of the placental or maternal peripheral blood) in the intervention group. According to the 14 trials included in the 2003 Cochrane database review[29], severe antenatal anaemia was less frequent in the group having received prophylaxis (RR = 0.62, 95% CI [0.50; 0.78]). In all studies but one[30] (Thailand: unstable malaria), there was an increase in birth weight and a reduction in LBW, particularly

Table 2 Antimalarial drugs currently used for prophylaxis in pregnant women

Drug	Dosage	Strengths	Limitations	Remarks
Chloroquine	300 mg, weekly	Well tolerated; inexpensive	Parasite resistance +; poor compliance	Used in trials in the 1980s and 1990s (Burkina Faso, Cameroon, Malawi, Papua New Guinea, etc.); present national policy in most of West Africa
Pyrimethamine	50 mg, monthly or 25 mg, weekly	Well tolerated; inexpensive	Parasite resistance ++	Used from the 1960s to the 1980s (Nigeria); now abandoned
Dapsone–pyrimethamine (prophylaxis)	Dapsone 100 mg and pyrimethamine 25 mg, fortnightly	Well tolerated; inexpensive	Parasite resistance ±; poor compliance; possibly teratogenic (if used in first trimester), cutaneous and haematological reactions	Used in the 1980s (The Gambia)
Sulfadoxine–pyrimethamine (intermittent treatment)	Sulfadoxine 1500 mg and pyrimethamine 75 mg, at each antenatal visit (max. three)	Well tolerated; inexpensive; good compliance	Parasite resistance ±; possibly teratogenic (if used in first trimester), cutaneous and haematological reactions	Used in trials in the 1990s (Malawi, Kenya); present national policy in several East African countries
Mefloquine	250 mg, weekly	Low parasite resistance (except in South East Asia)	Dizziness; possible effect on stillbirth; expensive	Used in trials in South East Asia and Malawi in the 1990s

++: high frequency; +: intermediate frequency; ±: low frequency.

British Medical Bulletin 2003;67

Table 3 Effect of chemoprophylaxis on maternal and fetal outcomes

Type of prophylaxis	Main study author(reference)	Country, year	Studied groups (n)	OR parasitaemia*[CI]	Difference in Hct**[CI]	OR anaemia***[CI]	Difference in birth weight**[CI]	OR LBW****[CI]
Pyrimethamine	Morley (27)	Nigeria, 1964	All (392)	0.13 [0.05; 0.33]	NC	NC	+157 [58; 256]	NC
			Primigravidae (55)		NC	NC	+190 [−80; 460]	NC
Dapsone–pyrimethamine	Greenwood (31)	Gambia, 1989	All (730)	0.38 [0.08; 1.78]	NC	NC	NC	NC
			Primigravidae (117)		+3.5 [0.7; 6.3]	NC	+146 [−5; 297]	NC
Chloroquine	Cot (32)	Burkina Faso, 1992	All (1148)	0.24 [0.16; 0.36]	+0.9 [0.2; 1.6]	0.85 [0.65; 1.11]	+6 [−47; 58]	0.99 [0.76; 1.29]
			Primigravidae (172)		+1.5 [−0.3; 3.3]	0.85 [0.43; 1.70]	+87 [−57; 221]	0.77 [0.49; 1.23]
Chloroquine	Cot (33)	Cameroon, 1995	Primigravidae (122)	0.47 [0.21; 1.04]	+2.0 [0.4; 3.6]	0.59 [0.25; 1.36]	+207 [34; 382]	0.38 [0.16; 0.89]
Mefloquine	Nosten (30)	Thailand, 1994	All (290)	0.13 [0.05; 0.32]	NC	NC	−80 [−182; 23]	1.39 [0.78; 2.48]
			Primigravidae (71)		+2.4 [1.0; 3.8]	NC		
Sulfadoxine–pyrimethamine	Shulman (34)	Kenya, 1999	All (1131)	0.10 [0.07; 0.16]	NC	0.54 [0.40; 0.74]	NC	NC
								NC

*Odds ratio for the risk of malarial infection (in the placenta: studies by Morley and Cot; in the peripheral blood: studies by Greenwood, Nosten and Shulman).

**Difference in haematocrit (%) or birth weight (g) between treated and control groups.

***Odds ratio for the risk of moderate anaemia (hct <30%: studies by Cot) or severe anaemia (Hb < 8 g/dl: study by Shulman).

****Odds ratio for the risk of low birth weight (< 2500 g).

in first and second pregnancies (RR = 0.49, 95% CI [0.36; 0.65]), and perinatal mortality seemed to be reduced (see also Table 3).

One of the main problems that appeared during the chemoprophylaxis trials is the growing resistance of the parasites to antimalarial treatments. Very soon after the first trial in Nigeria[27], it became obvious that pyrimethamine alone could no longer be used for prophylaxis, as it had lost a great deal of its usefulness. This is why subsequent intervention studies in Africa used dapsone–pyrimethamine or sulfadoxine–pyrimethamine (SP) combinations[31,34]. The same problem occurred (albeit to a lesser extent) with chloroquine. It is interesting to note that in our trial (1992) in Cameroon[33], although *in vivo* resistance attained 10% of the study population, there was still a substantial reduction in LBW in the treated group (Table 3). In areas of multiresistant malaria such as South East Asia, neither chloroquine nor SP combinations could be used, and mefloquine was administered to pregnant women initially[30].

Additionally, none of these drugs has been proven to be perfectly safe in pregnancy, except for chloroquine (Table 2). Questions remain about the teratogenic effects of folic acid antagonists (such as in the SP combinations), even if such risk appears to be significant only when treatment is given during the first trimester of pregnancy[35] (women usually do not start prophylaxis before the fourth or fifth month). There is also a possible association between the use of mefloquine and an increased risk of stillbirth[36]. Other drugs, such as tetracycline or halofantrine, are strictly forbidden during pregnancy. Quinine or artemisinin compounds cannot be used as prophylaxis because of their short half-life.

Another concern is the poor compliance generally observed with weekly or bi-monthly chemoprophylaxis, and ineffective blood levels induced from missing out one or several doses of anti-malarial drugs. In contrast, attendance at antenatal clinics (ANC) is generally good, and an important change in prevention strategies has occurred with the introduction of intermittent treatment with SP combinations in Malawi[37]. With this regimen, a single curative dose of three tablets is given two or three times (depending on the date of the first visit) at ANC visits (see Table 2). Though not evaluated as randomized trials (except one[34]), this regimen appears to be better accepted by pregnant women as well as being effective on placental infection, severe maternal anaemia and on incidence of LBW[34,37–39]. One of these studies[38] seems to indicate that placental malaria and LBW for HIV-positive women were improved through SP treatment at over two doses. If confirmed, this may have important consequences on prevention strategies, indicating that HIV-positive women should receive three SP doses at least.

Other protection measures

Vector control measures can act as a complement to prophylaxis to protect pregnant women against malaria. To our knowledge, only the effect of insecticide-treated bed nets (ITBNs) has been evaluated so far. The results are conflicting. Some studies (Thailand, The Gambia) indicate improvement in maternal anaemia, parasitaemia and LBW[40,41]. Others (Kenya, Ghana) did not show any noticeable effect of ITBNs on either the mother or the fetus[42,43].

Conclusions and future research

The administration of chemoprophylaxis during pregnancy has been proven to prevent placental malaria, maternal anaemia and LBW thanks to the randomized trials carried out in the 1980s and 1990s in highly endemic areas. However, poor compliance with weekly or bi-monthly regimens has led to the promotion of alternative strategies: intermittent treatment with SP combination given at ANC visits. These seem to be effective and more acceptable to pregnant women. This is national policy in several African countries and should be extended to areas where intense transmission of chloroquine-resistant *P. falciparum* occurs.

Whether to target interventions at high risk groups, such as primigravidae, secundigravidae or HIV-infected women when cost/benefit considerations are taken into account is not an easy question to answer. HIV and malaria co-infection seems to alter the normal pattern of increased susceptibility in primigravidae compared with multigravidae. It may be difficult to differentiate these groups when providing the intervention, as well as to exclude some women from receiving benefit. Therefore, the administration of SP intermittent treatment to all women may be the best strategy, when local resources permit it.

Some problems remain to be resolved. The decreasing efficiency of SP in HIV-positive pregnant women should be confirmed. Alternative drugs to SP should be developed, in case drug resistance intensifies.

These measures should be implemented along with other interventions such as the use of ITBNs, the systematic treatment of all malaria infections (which includes the use of quinine, mefloquine, or artemisinin derivatives), and more generally with other prenatal care programmes, including prevention of maternal anaemia and reduction in mother-to-child HIV transmission.

For the future, recent work on the property of parasitized erythrocytes to adhere to chondroitin sulphate A (CSA) expressed by the syncytiotrophoblast and then to accumulate in the placenta gives some hope for preventative or therapeutic interventions. This phenomenon is mediated by parasite variant surface antigens (VSA) expressed on the surface of infected erythrocytes[44]. Placental parasites bind to CSA, but not to the usual ligands of cytoadherence. The expression of a particular VSA by parasites binding to CSA in the placenta elicits variant-specific antibodies that are able to inhibit the cytoadherence of placental parasites to the human syncytiotrophoblast. The decreasing susceptibility to pregnancy-associated malaria with increasing parity is reflected in the acquisition of VSA_{CSA}-specific antibodies[45].

Recombinant CSA is efficient in inhibiting and reversing the placental cytoadherence of infected erythrocytes[46], and thus may constitute the basis of a causative therapy for placental malaria. VSA_{CSA}-specific antibodies react with placental parasites from all malaria endemic areas[47], and antibodies raised against the DBL3γ domain of PfEMP-1 (the major antigen constituting VSA) also inhibit the binding of placental parasites to CSA[48]. This represents a tremendous opportunity to develop a vaccine against pregnancy-associated malaria in the near future.

References

1 Clark HC. The diagnostic value of the placental blood film in aestivo-autumnal malaria. *J Exp Med* 1915; **22**: 427–45

2 McGregor IA. Epidemiology, malaria and pregnancy. *Am J Trop Med Hyg* 1984; **33**: 517–25

3 Menon R. Pregnancy and malaria. *Med J Malaysia* 1972; **27**: 115–9

4 Sholapurkar SL, Gupta AN, Mahajan RC. Clinical course of malaria in pregnancy—A prospective controlled study from India. *Trans R Soc Trop Med Hyg* 1988; **82**: 376–9

5 Nosten F, ter Kuile F, Maelankiri L, Decludt B, White NJ. Malaria during pregnancy in an area of unstable endemicity. *Trans R Soc Trop Med Hyg* 1991; **85**: 424–9

6 Cot M, Brutus L, Pinell V *et al*. Malaria prevention during pregnancy in unstable transmission areas: the highlands of Madagascar. *Trop Med Int Health* 2002; **7**: 565–72

7 Brabin B. *The Risks and Severity of Malaria in Pregnant Women*. Geneva: WHO (Applied Field Research in Malaria Reports No. 1), 1991

8 Menendez C. Malaria during pregnancy: A priority area of Malaria research and control. *Parasitol Today* 1995; **11**: 178–83

9 Steketee RW, Nahlen BL, Parise ME, Menedendez C. The burden of malaria in pregnancy in malaria-endemic areas. *Am J Trop Med Hyg* 2001; **64**: 28–35

10 Fleming AF. Tropical obstetrics and gynaecology. 1. Anaemia in pregnancy in tropical Africa. *Trans R Soc Trop Med Hyg* 1989; **83**: 441–8

11 Jackson DJ, Klee EB, Green SDR, Mokili JLK, Elton RA, Cutting WAM. Severe anaemia in pregnancy: a problem of primigravidae in rural Zaire. *Trans R Soc Trop Med Hyg* 1991; **85**: 829–32

12 Matteelli A, Donato F, Shein A *et al*. Malaria and anaemia in pregnant women in urban Zanzibar, Tanzania. *Ann Trop Med Parasitol* 1994; **88**: 475–83

13 Shulman CE, Graham WJ, Jilo H *et al*. Malaria is an important cause of anaemia in primigravidae: evidence for a district hospital in coastal Kenya. *Trans R Soc Trop Med Hyg* 1996; **90**: 535–9

14 Brabin BJ, Ginny M, Sapau J, Galme K, Paino J. Consequences of maternal anaemia on outcome of pregnancy in a malaria-endemic area in Papua New Guinea. *Ann Trop Med Parasitol* 1990; **84**: 11–24

15 Steer P, Ash Alama M, Wadsworth J, Welch A. Relation between maternal haemoglobin concentration and birth weight in different ethnic groups. *BMJ* 1995; **310**: 489–91

16   Fullerton WT, Turner AG. Exchange transfusion in the treatment of severe anaemia in pregnancy. *Lancet* 1962; Jan 13: 75–8

17   Brabin BJ, Verhoeff F. The contribution of malaria. In: McLean AB, Neilson JP (eds) *Maternal Morbidity and Mortality*. London: RCOG, 2002; 65–78

18   McDermott JM, Slutsker L, Steketee RW, Wirima JJ, Breman JG, Heymann DL. Prospective assessment of mortality among a cohort of pregnant women in rural Malawi. *Am J Trop Med Hyg* 1996; **55**: 66–70

19   Steketee RW, Wirima JJ, Hightower AW, Slutsker L, Heymann DL, Breman JG. The effect of malaria and malaria prevention in pregnancy on offspring birthweight, prematurity, and intra-uterine growth retardation in rural Malawi. *Am J Trop Med Hyg* 1996; **55**: 33–41

20   Redd SC, Wirima JJ, Steketee RW, Breman JG, Heymann DL. Transplacental transmission of *Plasmodium falciparum* in rural Malawi. *Am J Trop Med Hyg* 1996; **55**: 57–60

21   Kortmann HF. *Malaria and Pregnancy*. MD thesis: Drukkerij Elinkwijk, Utrecht, 1972

22   Steketee RW, Wirima JJ, Bloland PB *et al*. Impairment of a pregnant woman's acquired ability to limit *Plasmodium falciparum* by infection with human immunodeficiency virus type-1. *Am J Trop Med Hyg* 1996; **55**: 42–9

23   Verhoeff FH, Brabin BJ, Hart CA, Chimsuku L, Kazembe P, Broadhead RL. Increased preva-lence of malaria in HIV-infected pregnant women and its implications for malaria control. *Trop Med Int Health* 1999; **4**: 5–12

24   van Eijk AM, Ayisi JG, ter Kuile FO *et al*. HIV increases the risk of malaria in women of all gravidities in Kisumu, Kenya. *AIDS* 2003; **17**: 595–603

25   Rogerson SJ, Beeson JG. The placenta in malaria: mechanisms of infection, disease and foetal morbidity. *Ann Trop Med Parasitol* 1999; **93** (**Suppl. 1**): S35–42

26   Ayisi JG, van Eijk AM, ter Kuile FO *et al*. The effect of dual infection with HIV and malaria on pregnancy outcome in western Kenya. *AIDS* 2003; **17**: 585–94

27   Morley D, Woodland M, Cuthbertson WFJ. Controlled trial of pyrimethamine in pregnant women in an African village. *BMJ* 1964; **1**: 667–8

28   Garner P, Brabin B. A review of randomized controlled trials of routine antimalarial drug prophylaxis during pregnancy in endemic malarious areas. *Bull WHO* 1994; **72**: 89–99

29   Garner P, Gulmezoglu AM. Drugs for preventing malaria-related illness in pregnant women and death in the newborn (Cochrane Review). In: *The Cochrane Library, Issue 1, 2003*. Oxford: Update Software

30   Nosten F, ter Kuile F, Maelankiri L *et al*. Mefloquine prophylaxis prevents malaria during pregnancy: A double-blind, placebo-controlled study. *J Infect Dis* 1994; **169**: 595–603

31   Greenwood BM, Greenwood AM, Snow RW, Byass P, Bennett S, Hatib N'jie AB. The effects of malaria chemoprophylaxis given by traditional birth attendants on the course and outcome of pregnancy. *Trans R Soc Trop Med Hyg* 1989; **83**: 589–94

32   Cot M, Roisin A, Barro D, Yada A, Carnevale P, Breart G. Effect on birth weight of chloro-quine chemoprophylaxis during pregnancy: Results of a randomized trial. *Am J Trop Med Hyg* 1992; **46**: 21–7

33   Cot M, Le Hesran JY, Miailhes P, Esveld M, Etya'Ale D, Breart G. Increase of birth weight following a chloroquine chemoprophylaxis during first pregnancy: results of a randomized trial in Cameroon. *Am J Trop Med Hyg* 1995; **53**: 581–5

34   Shulman CE, Dorman EK, Cutts F *et al*. Intermittent sulphadoxine–pyrimethamine to prevent severe anaemia secondary to malaria in pregnancy: a randomised placebo-controlled trial. *Lancet* 1999; **353**: 632–6

35   Hernandez-Diaz S, Werler MM, Walker AM, Mitchell AA. Folic acid antagonists during pregnancy and the risk of birth defects. *N Engl J Med* 2000; **343**: 1608–14

36   Nosten F, Vincenti M, Simpson J *et al*. The effects of mefloquine treatment in pregnancy: A double-blind, placebo-controlled study. *Clin Infect Dis* 1999; **28**: 808–15

37   Schultz LJ, Steketee RW, Macheso A, Kazembe P, Chitsulo L, Wirima JJ. The efficacy of anti-malarial regimens containing sulfadoxine–pyrimethamine and/or chloroquine in preventing peripheral and placental *Plasmodium falciparum* infection among pregnant women in Malawi. *Am J Trop Med Hyg* 1994; **51**: 515–22

38   Parise ME, Ayisi JG, Nahlen BL *et al*. Efficacy of sulfadoxine–pyrimethamine for prevention of placental malaria in an area of Kenya with a high prevalence of malaria and human immuno-deficiency virus infection. *Am J Trop Med Hyg* 1998; **59**: 813–22

39 Verhoeff FH, Brabin BJ, Chimsuku L, Kazembe P, Russell WB, Broadhead RL. An evaluation of the effects of intermittent sulfadoxine–pyrimethamine treatment in pregnancy on parasite clearance and risk for low birthweight in rural Malawi. *Ann Trop Med Parasitol* 1998; **92:** 141–50

40 Dolan G, ter Kuile FO, Jacoutot V *et al.* Bed nets for the prevention of malaria and anaemia in pregnancy. *Trans R Soc Trop Med Hyg* 1993; **87:** 620–6

41 D'Alessandro U, Langerock P, Bennett S, Francis N, Cham K, Greenwood BM. The impact of a national impregnated bed net programme on the outcome of pregnancy in primigravidae in The Gambia. *Trans R Soc Trop Med Hyg* 1996; **90:** 487–92

42 Shulman CE, Dorman EK, Talisuna AO *et al.* A community randomised controlled trial of insecticide treated bednets for the prevention of malaria and anaemia among primigravid women on the Kenyan coast. *Trop Med Int Health* 1998; **3:** 197–204

43 Browne EN, Maude GH, Binka FN. The impact of insecticide-treated bednets on malaria and anaemia in pregnancy in Kassena-Nankana district, Ghana: a randomized controlled trial. *Trop Med Int Health* 2001; **6:** 667–76

44 Beeson JG, Brown GV. Pathogenesis of *Plasmodium falciparum* malaria: the roles of parasite adhesion and antigenic variation. *Cell Mol Life Sci* 2002; **59:** 258–71

45 Staalsoe T, Megnekou R, Fievet N *et al.* Acquisition and decay of antibodies to pregnancy-associated variant antigens on the surface of *Plasmodium falciparum* infected erythrocytes that are associated with protection against placental malaria. *J Infect Dis* 2001; **184:** 618–26

46 Chai W, Beeson JG, Kogelberg H, Brown GV, Lawson AM. Inhibition of adhesion of *Plasmodium falciparum*-infected erythrocytes by structurally defined hyaluronic acid dodecasaccharides. *Infect Immun* 2001; **69:** 420–5

47 Fried M, Nosten F, Brockman A, Brabin BJ, Duffy PE. Maternal antibodies block malaria. *Nature* 1998; **395:** 851–2

48 Lekana Douki JB, Traore B, Costa FT *et al.* Sequestration of *Plasmodium falciparum*-infected erythrocytes to chondroitin sulfate A, a receptor for maternal malaria: monoclonal antibodies against the native parasite ligand reveal pan-reactive epitopes in placental isolates. *Blood* 2002; **100:** 1478–83

Anaemia and micronutrient deficiencies

Nynke van den Broek

Liverpool School of Tropical Medicine, Liverpool, UK

Anaemia in pregnancy is a common and worldwide problem that deserves more attention. For many developing countries, prevalence rates of up to 75% are reported. Anaemia is frequently severe in these situations and can be expected to contribute significantly to maternal mortality and morbidity. After a discussion of definitions, screening for anaemia and prevalence, the relationship between anaemia and maternal mortality and morbidity will be reviewed. Micronutrient deficiency and especially iron deficiency is believed to be the main underlying cause for anaemia. More recently the role of vitamin A deficiency as a contributing factor to anaemia has also been examined. The difficulties of assessment of micronutrient sufficiency or deficiency in pregnancy are described, as is the interaction between infection and micronutrient deficiency states.

Definitions

Correspondence to:
Dr N van den Broek,
Senior Lecturer
Reproductive Health,
Liverpool School of
Tropical Medicine,
Pembroke Place,
Liverpool L3 5QA, UK.
E-mail: vdbroek@liv.ac.uk

As a result of the normal physiological changes in pregnancy, plasma volume expands by 46–55%, whereas red-cell volume expands by 18–25%[1,2]. The resulting haemodilution has, perhaps wrongly, been termed 'physiological anaemia of pregnancy'. There are in fact insufficient data to give accurate physiological limits for the expected haemodilution. In most published studies, the mean minimum normal haemoglobin in healthy pregnant women living at sea level is 11.0–12.0 g/dl. The mean minimum by WHO criteria is taken to be 11.0 g/dl in the first half of pregnancy and 10.5 g/dl in the second half of pregnancy[3,4]. In the only well-conducted longitudinal study that could be found of the 'hydraemia' of pregnancy in iron-replete healthy pregnant women, 10.4 g/dl was the lowest recorded value[5].

Anaemia in pregnancy is further divided into mild anaemia ([Hb] 10.0–10.9 g/dl), moderate anaemia ([Hb] 7.0–9.9 g/dl) and severe anaemia ([Hb]<7.0 g/dl)[4]. The definition of severe anaemia in the published literature, however, varies and this may also be defined as [Hb]<8.0 g/dl. There is discussion in the literature about the relevance of the various cut-off points, whether different cut-off points should be used for different populations[5–8] and the need to adjust for populations living at high altitude[9].

Screening

An accepted standard of practice is that all women have at least one haemoglobin measurement during the course of pregnancy. This is usually carried out by electronic (automated) counter. In many developing countries, these methods are not available at Health Centre level and may not be available even at tertiary level. Either screening for anaemia may not be carried out at all or assessment of whether a pregnant woman is anaemic or not may be limited to inspection of the conjunctiva by the nurse or midwife for the presence of pallor during antenatal visits.

There are few published papers reporting on the accuracy of screening for anaemia using clinical inspection of conjunctiva in pregnant women. In a large study conducted in women attending a rural antenatal clinic, sensitivity was 33.2% and 39.7% for haemoglobin values of ≤11.0 and ≤10.0 g/dl, respectively. Values obtained were better for the lower range of haemoglobin values but did not exceed 62.1%[10]. A study from Mozambique reported a sensitivity of 31.5%, with anaemia defined as a packed cell volume ≤30[11]. In a smaller study from Kenya, examination of the conjunctiva was reported to have 62–69% sensitivity for detecting severe anaemia ([Hb] < 7.0 g/dl) in a study population with a high incidence of severe anaemia (16%)[12]. Substantial interobserver variability has also been reported[13,14]. Even when used in combination with a conjunctival—or anaemia—recognition card, sensitivity remains low except when anaemia is severe[15,16].

In the absence of a functioning automated (Coulter) counter, several alternative methods for measurement of haemoglobin concentration are available[17]. A relatively expensive but simple to use portable haemoglobin meter (HemoCue) has been evaluated and found to have a sensitivity of between 80% and 97% and a specificity of between 79% and 99% depending on the cut-off points for haemoglobin concentration used[10,18–20]. Another method which has been studied in antenatal clinic settings is the copper sulphate method[21–24]. This method relies on the preparation and availability of a solution of copper sulphate of known specific gravity. There is a fixed range of haemoglobin values for which a blood sample can be tested, *e.g.* [Hb] < 8.0 g/dl or < 10.0 g/dl.

In response to the need for a simple, cheap and accurate method for the estimation of haemoglobin concentration, a new Colour Scale was recently developed by the WHO[25] which is similar to the Talquist[26] scale and consists of a card with 6 colour standards corresponding to the colour of bloodstains of various haemoglobin concentrations (range 4.0–14.0 g/dl). Assessment in an antenatal population with high prevalence of anaemia by comparison with Coulter counter measurements gave sensitivities of 75.4% and 81.6% for cut-off points of [Hb] <11.0 and <10.0 g/dl, respectively. Specificity was 47.2% and 45.3%, respectively, but improved to 76.4% for [Hb] < 8.0 g/dl and 98.5% for [Hb] < 6.0 g/dl. The sensitivity of the WHO Colour Scale as a screening tool to detect anaemia was consistently better than if conjunctival inspection was used for screening[10].

Prevalence

It has been estimated that over half the pregnant women in the world have a haemoglobin level indicative of anaemia. In industrialized countries, anaemia in pregnancy occurs in less than 20% of women. This does, however, still reach the level of public health significance (≥ 10%). Published rates of prevalence for developing countries range from 35% to 72% for Africa, 37–75% for Asia and 37–52% for Latin America[27]. Not only is anaemia common, it is often severe. From the published reports available, it can be estimated that 2–7% of pregnant women have values < 7.0 g/dl, and, probably 15–20% < 8.0 g/dl. Those authors who publish their range of haemoglobin values not infrequently report on patients with values well below 5.0 g/dl[28–30]. Up-to-date information from many countries is, however, still scanty; the few published studies often describe small sample sizes and are usually from hospital-based populations. There is a lack of data from rural areas. It has been suggested that the prevalence of anaemia may depend on the season, increasing in relation to malaria transmission in the wet season or in relation to increased food shortage at the end of the dry season, but published prevalence rates rarely reflect measurements performed all year round.

In 1993, the World Bank[31] ranked anaemia as the eighth leading cause of disease in girls and women in developing countries. Although anaemia is assumed to be less common in non-pregnant women, there is a lack of data on the prevalence of anaemia in this population group. Studies are also needed to assess the association between anaemia in pregnancy and pre-pregnancy haemoglobin levels.

Anaemia and maternal mortality and morbidity

Each year more than 500,000 women die from pregnancy-related causes, 99% of these in developing countries[32]. Estimates of maternal mortality resulting from anaemia range from 34/100,000 live births in Nigeria to as high as 194/100,000 in Pakistan[4,27]. In combination with obstetric haemorrhage, anaemia is estimated to be responsible for 17–46% of cases of maternal death[33–35]. A review of symptoms associated with maternal deaths in Bangladesh led researchers to conclude that anaemia had played a secondary role in nearly all cases[36].

Anaemia is probably a chronic rather than acute condition in many cases. There is a resulting compensatory shift of the oxygen dissociation curve to the right. Thus, women with very low haemoglobin concentrations may be seen in the antenatal period without the expected overt symptoms of cardiac failure. They will, however, easily become tired by any form of physical activity and may decompensate, *e.g.* as a result of labour. Should any adverse event such as bleeding occur, their risk of death is high.

The available data on the association between anaemia and maternal survival are limited and there are serious methodological flaws in most of the studies, as pointed out by Rush[37] in his excellent review. It must be noted that pregnancy outcome will also be related to the underlying causes of anaemia, *e.g.* HIV, iron deficiency, recurrent antepartum haemorrhage, *etc*. Most of the published studies report on outcome for hospital-based patients. In developing countries, this is rarely representative of the population as a whole. In particular, conclusions about association or causality drawn from a single measurement during delivery in hospital must be considered flawed. In many cases, haemoglobin concentration may have been measured only because of, for instance, a prior history of bleeding, fever or suspected malaria, which may be the reason for referral to the hospital in the first place.

It must also be noted that there are currently no agreed international standards or sets of criteria for attributing death to anaemia. It is in fact often difficult to establish accurately the cause of death in situations where clinical information is incomplete and data collection is not standardized. Thus, in many cases, the only two laboratory tests that may have been available to clinicians could be a haemoglobin concentration and a peripheral blood slide for malaria parasitaemia. Death from anaemia may sound better than death from haemorrhage, in that the latter could be perceived as the result of the health facility's inability to provide adequate care. Finally, level of access to emergency obstetric care and in particular to blood transfusion and the quality and speed of care received are of prime determining importance. Thus, a study from Indonesia[38] illustrated the much higher risk of maternal death in anaemic women from rural areas than from urban areas, possibly as a result of problems with timely access to obstetric care.

Morbidity resulting from anaemia is similarly difficult to establish. Diminished work capacity and physical performance have been reported as a result of anaemia[39,40].

Iron deficiency anaemia leads to abnormalities in host defence and neurological dysfunction[41,42]. Increased risks of premature labour[43–45] and low birth weight[43,46,47] have also been reported in association with anaemia in pregnancy. Both are common problems in developing countries and contribute significantly to high perinatal mortality. However, most published work on this comes from industrialized countries where anaemia is much less of a problem and much less severe in nature. Confounding factors such as poverty, poor antenatal clinic attendance and recurrent infection, which can result in low birth weight and prematurity, are seldom examined at the same time. Further research on the effect of anaemia *per se* on birth weight and prematurity is therefore necessary to establish a clear causal relationship.

Micronutrients and pregnancy

Vitamins and minerals are referred to collectively as the 'micronutrients'. The micronutrient deficiencies which are thought to be of the greatest public health significance globally are iron deficiency, vitamin A deficiency and iodine deficiency. Both iron deficiency and vitamin A deficiency can result in anaemia. Dietary inadequacy is thought to be the major cause for vitamin A and iron deficiency.

Iron deficiency

Iron is obtained in the form of non-haem iron from vegetables and as haem iron from meat. Haem iron is absorbed about two to three times better than non-haem iron. A small amount of haem iron in the diet will improve absorption of non-haem iron and thus the diet composition is an important determinant of the amount of iron actually absorbed. Iron is stored in the reticulo-endothelial system as ferritin and haemosiderin. Iron is a component of haemoglobin and iron deficiency ultimately leads to defective erythropoiesis and anaemia.

Pregnant women are particularly vulnerable to iron deficiency as a result of the increased demand for iron. The requirements for iron during pregnancy have been estimated at a total of about 1000 mg[1,48]. In response to pregnancy, iron absorption is increased[48,49].

The marked physiological changes that occur in pregnancy influence the laboratory measurements used to evaluate iron status. The expansion of plasma volume, increase in erythropoiesis and increased demand of the fetoplacental unit for iron occur throughout gestation and can vary markedly between individuals. The resulting changes in serum levels of biochemical markers for iron status make it necessary to re-define cut-off values for the diagnosis of iron deficiency in pregnancy[50]. Serum ferritin is the most frequently used indicator of iron status.

The range of values for serum ferritin found in non-anaemic individuals is 12–300 µg/l. In the presence of anaemia, values of <20 µg/l are commonly taken as evidence of iron deficiency[51]. However, patients with levels of up to 37 µg/l have been shown to have absent marrow haemosiderin[52]. In pregnancy, serum ferritin is lower and mean values are close to the iron deficient range[53]. More recently, the measurement of serum transferrin receptors and the serum transferrin receptor/ferritin ratio have been proposed as new indices of iron deficiency[54,55]. Receptor synthesis is up-regulated in iron deprived tissues. It can be argued that assessment of iron status at the tissue level is of more functional importance when examining the effects of iron depletion on the body than an assessment of stores.

Because of the increase in absorption during pregnancy coupled with the mobilization of iron stores, if women of childbearing age have enough iron stores to cope with the demands of pregnancy this could be sufficient and iron supplements may not be necessary. However, if iron stores are low, supplementation may be necessary or indicated. Provision of routine iron supplementation to pregnant women who do not have evidence of iron deficiency and have Hb levels > 10 g/dl has been shown to have a positive effect on women's iron status. The prevalence of low pre-delivery haemoglobin and low haemoglobin at 6 weeks post partum is reduced. There is more stainable iron in the bone marrow with higher serum iron and ferritin levels[56].

Vitamin A deficiency

Vitamin A is a fat soluble vitamin which is obtained from the diet as preformed vitamin A (retinal) and from some of the carotenoid pigments in food that can be cleaved in the body to give retinol. Preformed vitamin A occurs naturally only in animals and the richest dietary sources are liver, fish oils and dairy products. Between 25 and 35% of the dietary vitamin A will come from carotenoids mainly from plant foods such as carrots and dark leafy vegetables. Carotenoids can be converted to vitamin A in the liver where vitamin A is stored. Absorption from plant sources is thought to be low and animal sources may be needed to achieve adequate levels. The digestion and absorption of vitamin A are also closely linked with lipid absorption and therefore low dietary fat intake may interfere with vitamin A absorption.

Vitamin A deficiency is thought to be common in many developing countries. Much of the work on prevalence has been in children and there is comparatively little information about the occurrence in pregnancy. Estimates of the number of people at risk from vitamin A deficiency are often approximations but it is thought that there is a significant problem in most parts of Africa, South and South East Asia and areas of Latin America and the Western Pacific[57]. In case of marginal vitamin A deficiency, the extra demands made by pregnancy could be expected to result in vitamin A deficiency symptoms such as night blindness.

Assessment of vitamin A status in pregnancy is commonly by measurement of serum retinol. However, serum retinol levels are under strict homeostatic control and not a good measure for individual vitamin A status. Dose response tests have recently been developed which assess vitamin A stores in the liver and this is a more accurate method of assessment[58,59]. In pregnancy, as a result of the physiological changes described above, serum retinol levels have been shown to drop below non-pregnancy concentrations[60].

Vitamin A is believed to be essential for normal embryogenesis, haematopoiesis, growth and epithelial differentiation. In pregnancy, extra vitamin A is required for growth and tissue maintenance in the fetus, for providing it with reserves and for maternal metabolism. Basal requirements in pregnancy are 370 µg per day, which increase during lactation to 450 µg per day.

On the other hand, a relationship has been suggested between the incidence of birth defects and high vitamin A intakes during pregnancy with an apparent threshold of 10,000 IU per day[61–63]. However daily doses of up to 10,000 IU or weekly doses of 25,000 IU after day 60 of pregnancy are safe, especially in areas where vitamin A deficiency is common[61].

Vitamin A is essential for haematopoiesis. A diet devoid of vitamin A results in decreased haemoglobin levels[64]. Antenatal supplementation with both iron and vitamin A was shown to reduce anaemia prevalence in a study from Indonesia[65] but other studies conducted in sub-Saharan Africa were not able to obtain the same positive result[66]. The mechanism whereby vitamin A supplementation could improve haemoglobin and iron status has not been fully elucidated but it has been suggested that vitamin A is required for the mobilization and utilization of iron for haemoglobin synthesis[67]. An anti-infective role has also been suggested as infection is known to be associated with decreased serum iron levels, suppressed erythropoiesis and lower haemoglobin concentration[68]. An important and large study from Nepal has recently generated discussion about the role of vitamin A in the possible reduction in maternal mortality[69]. A clear biological explanation could not be given and anaemia was not studied as an outcome in this trial. Further trials are currently under way to address these issues. Currently, WHO recommends routine vitamin A supplementation during pregnancy or at any time during lactation in areas with endemic vitamin A deficiency (where night blindness occurs)[61].

Micronutrient deficiency and anaemia

Relatively few studies have comprehensively assessed the aetiological factors responsible for anaemia in pregnancy and this is especially so for developing countries where anaemia is more prevalent and more severe and likely to have a greater contribution to maternal mortality and morbidity than in industrialized countries. This is probably for three main reasons. (1) The lack of adequate diagnostic facilities in many institutions in developing countries. (2) The frequent complexity of the aetiological pattern, such that, for example, infection and nutritional deficiency coexist. (3) The relative contribution of each aetiological factor can be difficult to assess in pregnancy when maternal physiological changes alter the parameters used to diagnose deficiency or sufficiency.

Chemical measurements of iron status are influenced by inflammation, and there is a lack of clearly defined and validated cut-off points for the diagnosis of deficiency in these circumstances[70]. Evaluation of suitably stained bone marrow aspirates may then be necessary to provide meaningful results[71].

Despite the lack of stringent criteria and definitional problems, pregnancy anaemia in sub-Saharan Africa is most often believed to be the result of nutritional deficiencies, especially iron deficiency[72,73]. Folate deficiency has been described in West Africa[74]. Studies from Indonesia indicate that vitamin A deficiency may contribute to anaemia in pregnancy[65]. Vitamin B12 deficiency was found to be an unrecognized but important cause of anaemia in Zimbabwe[75]. It must be noted that micronutrient deficiencies are often studied in isolation but in actual fact are very likely to occur together and in many cases there is a multiple micronutrient deficiency state.

In many developing countries, it is difficult to meet daily nutrient requirements with diet alone especially for pregnant women. Animal products and fats are often relatively expensive and in addition, there may be food taboos which influence dietary intake in pregnancy. The benefit of multiple micronutrient supplements is therefore being considered[76].

Although the contribution of malaria is generally acknowledged, the role of other chronic infections has been discussed[77] but not extensively studied in pregnant women. In the last decade, HIV infection has become more prevalent and it must now be considered a possible aetiological factor[30,78]. A recent study from Malawi illustrates the complex interaction between multi-micronutrient deficiency and infection[71].

Thus, possible aetiological factors responsible for anaemia are multiple and their relative contributions can be expected to vary by geographical area, as well as by season. Knowledge of the relative importance of different causes should form the basis for intervention strategies.

Key points

- In many areas of the world, as many as 75% of women are anaemic during pregnancy by WHO standards ([Hb] < 11.0 g/dl). Many have severe anaemia ([Hb] < 7.0 g/dl or < 8.0 g/dl). It is not known whether most women enter pregnancy already anaemic or whether anaemia develops primarily during pregnancy. Detection of anaemia often relies solely on conjunctival inspection, which is probably insufficient. The introduction of cheap but accurate screening tools should be encouraged.

- There is a lack of studies measuring haemoglobin levels prospectively before and during pregnancy with assessment of maternal mortality and morbidity. Thus, it is not possible to indicate which level of haemoglobin is particularly associated with adverse outcome. However, on the basis of the available evidence, it seems reasonable to assume that the risk of maternal mortality in developing countries is increased, especially with severe anaemia.

- In many pregnant women, anaemia is probably caused by a combination of disease including both micronutrient deficiency and infection. The complex pattern of interaction between the two requires further study. Haemoglobin concentration should perhaps be regarded as a 'marker of morbidity' in these situations.

References

1 Letsky EA. The haematological system. In: Hytten F, Chamberlain G, Broughton Pipkin F (eds) *Clinical Physiology in Obstetrics*. Oxford: Blackwell Scientific Publications, 1998; 71–110

2 Letsky EA. Blood volume, haematinics, anaemia. In: de Swiet M (ed) *Medical Disorders in Obstetric Practice*, 3rd edn. Oxford: Blackwell Science, 1995; 33–70

3 World Health Organization. *Nutritional Anaemias*. Technical report series no. 503. Geneva: WHO; 1972

4 World Health Organization. *Prevention and Management of Severe Anaemia in Pregnancy*. Geneva: WHO; 1993

5 Leeuw NKM, de, Lowenstein L, Hsieh YS. Iron deficiency anaemia and hydraemia in normal pregnancy. *Medicine Baltimore* 1966; **45**: 291–315

6 Johnson-Spear MA, Yip R. Hemoglobin difference between black and white women with comparable iron status: justification for race-specific anaemia criteria. *Am J Clin Nutr* 1994; **60**: 117–21

7 Dallman PR, Barr GD, Allen AM. Hemoglobin concentration in white, black and oriental children: is there a need for separate criteria in screening for anemia. *Am J Clin Nutr* 1978; **31**: 377–80

8 Berti P, Leonard WR. The merits of race-specific standards. *Am J Clin Nutr* 1994; **60**: 616

9 Berger J, Aguayo VM, San Miguel JL, Lujan C, Tellez W, Traissac MS. Definition and prevalence of anemia in Bolivian women of childbearing age living at high altitudes: the effect of iron-folate supplementation. *Nutr Rev* 1997; **55**: 247–56

10 van den Broek NR, Ntonya C, Mhango E, White SA. Diagnosing anemia in pregnancy in rural clinics: assessing the potential of the Haemoglobin Colour Scale. *Bull World Health Organ* 1999; **77**: 15–21

11 Liljestrand J, Bergstrom S. The value of conjunctival pallor in the diagnosis of pregnancy anaemia in Mozambique. *J Obstet Gynaecol East Centr Afr* 1992; **10**: 45–6

12 Shulman CE, Levene M, Morison L, Dorman E, Peshu N, Marsh K. Screening for severe anaemia in pregnancy in Kenya, using pallor examination and self-reported morbidity. *Trans R Soc Trop Med Hyg* 2001; **95**: 250–5

13 Gjorup T, Bugge PM, Hendriksen C, Jensen AM. A critical evaluation of the clinical diagnosis of anemia. *Am J Epidemiol* 1986; **124**: 657–65

14 Sanchez-Carrillo CI. Bias due to conjunctiva hue and the clinical assessment of anemia. *J Clin Epidemiol* 1989; **42**: 751–4

15 Sanchez-Carillo CI, de Jesus Ramirez-Sanchez T, Zambrana-Castenada M, Selwyn BJ. Test of a non-invasive instrument for measuring haemoglobin concentration. *Int J Technol Assess Health Care* 1989; **5**: 659–67

16 Ghosh S, Mohan M. Screening for anaemia. *Lancet* 1978; **1**: 823

17 United States Agency for International Development. *PATH—Program for Appropriate Technology in Health. Anemia Detection in Health Services. Guidelines for Program Managers.* Washington, DC: USAID; 1996

18 van den Broek NR, Kayira E, White SA, Medina A, Neilson JP, Molyneux ME. The accuracy of measuring haemoglobin concentration using a HemoCue haemoglobinometer: comparison with an automated method; In press

19 Neville RG. Evaluation of portable hemoglobinometer in general practice. *BMJ (Clin Res Edn)* 1987; **294**: 1263–5

20 Hudson-Thomas M, Bingham KC, Simmons WK. An evaluation of the HemoCue for measuring haemoglobin in field studies in Jamaica. *Bull World Health Organ* 1994; **72**: 423–6

21 Politzer WM, Myburgh WM, van der Merwe JF. Haemoglobin estimation—reliability of the copper sulphate specific gravity v. the cyanhaemoglobin colorimetric method. *S Afr Med J* 1988; **73**: 111–2

22 Pistorius LR, Funk M, Pattinson RC, Howarth GR. Screening for anaemia in pregnancy with copper sulfate densitometry. *Int J Gynaecol Obstet* 1996; **52**: 3–36

23 Kegels G, Cornelis G, Mangelschots E, Van Brabant R, van Lerberghe W. Haemoglobin and packed cell volume measurement: the reliability of some simple techniques for use in surveys or rural hospitals. *Ann Soc Belg Med Trop* 1984; **64**: 413–9

24 Wilkinson D, Sach ME. Cost-effective on-site screening for anaemia in pregnancy in primary clinics. *S Afr Med J* 1997; **87**: 463–5

25 Stott GJ, Lewis SM. A simple and reliable method for estimating haemoglobin. *Bull World Health Organ* 1995; **73**: 369–73

26 Tallqvist TW. Méthode protique d'évaluation directe de la quantité d'hémoglobine du sang. *Arch Gen Med* 1900; **3**: 421–5

27 World Health Organization. *The Prevalence of Anaemia in Women: A Tabulation of Available Information.* Geneva: WHO, 1992

28 van den Broek NR, Rogerson SJ, Mhango CG, Kambala B, White SA, Molyneux ME. Anaemia in pregnancy in southern Malawi: prevalence and risk factors. *Br J Obstet Gynaecol* 2000; **107**: 445–51

29 Bergsjo P, Seha Am, Ole-King'ori N. Haemoglobin concentration in pregnant women. Experience from Moashi—Tanzania. *Acta Obstet Gynecol Scand* 1996; **75**: 241–4

30 Fleming AF. The aetiology of severe anaemia in pregnancy in Ndola, Zambia. *Ann Trop Med Parasitol* 1989; **83**: 37–49

31 World Bank. *World Development Report: Investing in Health.* New York: Oxford University Press, 1993; 1–329

32 World Health Organization. *Maternal Mortality Ratios and Rates.* Geneva: WHO, 1996

33 World Bank, WHO, UNFPA. Preventing the tragedy of maternal deaths. A report on the International Safe Motherhood Conference Nairobi, Kenya, 1987. Geneva: WHO.

34 Harrison KA. Maternal mortality. *Trans R Soc Trop Med Hyg* 1989; **83**: 449–53

35 Harrison KA. Severity of anaemia and operative mortality and morbidity. *Lancet* 1988; June 18: 1392

36 Alauddin M. Maternal mortality in rural Bangladesh. The Tangail District. *Stud Fam Plann* 1986; **17**: 13–21

37 Rush D. Nutrition and maternal mortality in the developing world. *Am J Clin Nutr* 2000; **72** (**Suppl.**): 212–40

38 Chi I, Agoestina T, Harbin J. Maternal mortality at twelve teaching hospitals in Indonesia: an epidemiologic analysis. *Int J Gynaecol Obstet* 1992; **39:** 87–92

39 Viteri FE, Torun B. Anaemia and physical work capacity. In: Garby L (ed) *Clinics in Haematology,* vol. **3,** WB Saunders, 1974; 609–26

40 Hallberg L, Scrimshaw NS. *Iron Deficiency and Work Performance.* International Nutritional Anemia Consultative Group, 1981

41 Cook JD, Lynch SR. The liabilities of iron deficiency. *Blood* 1986; **68:** 803–9

42 Dallman PR. Iron deficiency and the immune response. *Am J Clin Nutr* 1987; **46:** 329–34

43 Garn SM, Ridella SA, Petzold AS, Falkner F. Maternal hematologic levels and pregnancy outcomes. *Semin Perinatol* 1981; **5:** 155–62

44 Klebanoff MA, Shiono PH, Selby JV, Trachtenberg AI, Graubard BI. Anemia and spontaneous preterm birth. *Am J Obstet Gynecol* 1991; **164:** 59–63

45 Allen LH. Iron-deficiency anemia increases risk of preterm delivery. *Nutr Rev* 51; **2:** 49–52

46 Mitchell MC, Lerner E. Maternal hematologic measures and pregnancy outcome. *J Am Diet Assoc* 1992; **92:** 484–6

47 Harrison KA, Ibeziako PA. Maternal anaemia and fetal birth weight. *J Obstet Gynaecol Br Cwlth* 1973; **80:** 798–804

48 Hallberg L. Iron balance in pregnancy and lactation. In: Fomon SJ, Zlotkin S (eds) *Nutritional Anemias,* Nestle Nutrition Workshop Series, vol. **30,** 1992; 13–28

49 Barrett JFR, Whitaker PG, Williams JG, Lind T. Absorption of non-haem iron in food during normal pregnancy. *BMJ* 1994; **309:** 79–82

50 van den Broek NR, Letsky EA, White SA, Shenkin A. Iron status in pregnant women: which parameters are valid? *Br J Haematol* 1998; **103:** 817–24

51 Cook JD. Iron deficiency anaemia. *Baillière's Clin Haematol* 1994; **7:** 787–804

52 Lipschitz DA, Cook JD, Finch CA. A clinical evaluation of serum ferritin as an index of iron stores. *N Engl J Med* 1974; **290:** 1213–6

53 Hallberg L. Prevention of iron deficiency. *Baillière's Clin Haematol* 1994; **7:** 805–14

54 Flowers CH, Skikne BS, Covell AM, Cook JD. The clinical measurement of serum transferrin receptor. *J Lab Clin Med* 1989; **114:** 368–77

55 Skikne BS, Flowers CH, Cook JD. Serum transferrin receptor: A quantitative measure of tissue iron deficiency. *Blood* 1990; **75:** 1870–6

56 Mahomed K. Iron supplementation in pregnancy (Cochrane Review). In: *The Cochrane Library, Issue 4, 2002.* Oxford: Update Software

57 WHO. *Global Prevalence of Vitamin A Deficiency. Micronutrient Deficiency Information System.* WHO/NUT/95. Geneva: WHO, 1995

58 WHO. *Indicators for Assessing Vitamin A Deficiency and Their Application in Monitoring and Evaluating Intervention Programs.* WHO/NUT/94.1 Geneva: WHO, 1994

59 Tanumidhardjo SA, Suharno D, Parmaesih D *et al.* Application of the modified relative dose response test to pregnant women for assessing Vitamin A status. *Eur J Clin Nutr* 1992; **49:** 897–903

60 Hytten FE. Nutrition. In: Hytten FE, Chamberlain G (eds) *Clinical Physiology in Obstetrics.* Oxford: Blackwell Publications, 1991: 163–93

61 WHO. *Safe Vitamin A Dosage During Pregnancy and Lactation. Recommendations and a Report of a Consultation.* WHO/NUT/98. Geneva: WHO, 1998

62 Mills JL, Simpson JL, Cunningham GC, Comley MA, Rhoads GG. Vitamin A and birth defects. *Am J Obstet Gynecol* 1997; **177:** 31–6

63 Rothman KJ, Moore LL, Singer MR, Nguyen UDT, Mannino S, Milunsky A. Teratogenicity of high Vitamin A intake. *N Engl J Med* 1995; **333:** 1367–73

64 Hodges RE, Sauberlich HE, Canham JE *et al.* Hematopoietic studies in Vitamin A deficiency. *Am J Clin Nutr* 1978; **31:** 876–85

65 Suharno D, West CE, Muhilal, Karyadi D, Hautvast GAJ. Supplementation with vitamin A and iron for nutritional anaemia in pregnant women in West Java, Indonesia. *Lancet* 1993; **342:** 1325–8

66 van den Broek NR, Kulier R, Gulmezoglu AM, Villar J. Vitamin A supplementation during pregnancy (Cochrane Review). In: *The Cochrane Library, Issue 5, 2003.* Oxford: Update Software

67 Bloem MW, Wedel M, van Agtmaal EJ, Speek AJ, Soawakontha S, Schreurs WHP. Vitamin A intervention: short term effects of a single oral massive dose on iron metabolism. *Am J Clin Nutr* 1990; **51**: 76–9

68 Thurnham DI. Vitamin A and haematopoiesis. *Lancet* 1993; **342**: 1312–3

69 West KP, Kratz J, Khatry SK *et al.* Double blind randomised trial of low dose supplements with Vitamin A or beta carotene on mortality related to pregnancy in Nepal. The NNIPS-Study Group. *BMJ* 1999; **318**: 570–5

70 Cook JD, Baynes RD, Skikne BS. Iron deficiency and the measurement of iron status. *Nutr Res Rev* 1992; **5**: 189–202

71 van den Broek NR. The aetiology of anaemia in pregnancy in West Africa. *Trop Doct* 1996; **26**: 5–7

72 Baker SJ, DeMaeyer EM. Nutritional anemia: its understanding and control with special reference to the work of the World Health Organization. *Am J Clin Nutr* 1979; **32**: 368–417

73 DeMaeyer EM, Adiels-Tegman M. The prevalence of anaemia in the world. *World Health Stat Q* 1985; **38**: 302–16

74 Fleming AF. A Study of Anaemia in Pregnancy in Ibadan, Western Nigeria with Special Reference to Folic Acid Deficiency. Thesis: Cambridge: Cambridge University, 1968

75 Savage D, Gangaidzo I, Lindenbaum J, Kiire C, Mukiibi JM, Moyo A *et al.* Vitamin B12 deficiency is the primary cause of megaloblastic anaemia in Zimbabwe. *Br J Haematol* 1994; **86**: 844–50

76 Huffman Sl, Baker J, Shumann MA, Zehner ER. *The Case for Promoting Multiple Vitamin/Mineral Supplements for Women of Reproductive Age in Developing Countries. The Linkages Project*. Washington, DC: Population Services International, 1998

77 Yip R, Dallman PR. The roles of inflammation and iron deficiency as causes of anemia. *Am J Clin Nutr* 1988; **48**: 1295–300

78 van den Broek NR, White SA, Neilson JP. The association between asymptomatic human immunodeficiency virus infection and the prevalence and severity of anemia in pregnant Malawian women. *Am J Trop Med Hyg* 1998; **59**: 1004–7

Pre-eclampsia and the hypertensive disorders of pregnancy

Lelia Duley

Resource Centre for Randomised Trials, Institute of Health Sciences, Headington, Oxford, UK

Pre-eclampsia is a multisystem disorder, of unknown aetiology, usually associated with raised blood pressure and proteinuria. Although outcome for most women and their babies is good, it remains a major cause of morbidity and mortality. A wide range of interventions for prevention and treatment of pre-eclampsia have been evaluated in randomized trials. This evidence provides the basis for a rational approach to care. Overall, there is insufficient evidence for any firm conclusion about the effects of any aspect of diet or lifestyle during pregnancy. Antiplatelet agents are associated with a 19% reduction in the risk of pre-eclampsia (relative risk 0.81; 95% CI 0.75, 0.88), a 7% reduction in the risk of preterm birth (RR 0.93; 95% CI 0.89, 0.98), a 16% reduction in the risk of stillbirth or neonatal death (RR 0.84; 95% CI 0.74, 0.96) and an 8% reduction in the risk of a small for gestational age baby (RR 0.92; 95% CI 0.85, 1.00). For mild to moderate hypertension, trials evaluating bed rest are too small for reliable conclusions about the potential benefits and hazards. Antihypertensive agents halve the risk of progression to severe hypertension (RR 0.52; 95% CI 0.41, 0.64), but with no clear effect on pre-eclampsia (RR 0.99; 95% CI 0.84, 1.18), or any other substantive outcome. For severe hypertension, there is no good evidence that one drug is any better than another. Plasma volume expansion for severe pre-eclampsia seems unlikely to be beneficial, although the trials are small. The optimum timing of delivery for pre-eclampsia before 34 weeks is unclear. Magnesium sulphate more than halves the risk of eclampsia (RR 0.41; 95% CI 0.29, 0.58) and probably reduces the risk of maternal death (RR 0.54; 95% CI 0.26, 1.10). It is also the drug of choice for treatment of eclampsia.

Introduction

Correspondence to: Lelia Duley, Resource Centre for Randomised Trials, Institute of Health Sciences, Old Road, Headington, Oxford OX3 7LF, UK. E-mail: rcrt@ndm.ox.ac.uk

Pre-eclampsia is a multisystem disorder of unknown aetiology, unique to pregnancy. Women with pre-eclampsia usually develop raised blood pressure and proteinuria, but the condition is also associated with abnormalities of the coagulation system, disturbed liver function, renal failure and cerebral ischaemia[1]. It complicates an estimated 2–8% of pregnancies and is a major cause of maternal morbidity, perinatal death and premature delivery, although outcome for most women is good. Eclampsia, the occurrence of one or more convulsions superimposed on the syndrome of pre-eclampsia, occurs less frequently, complicating between 1 in 100–1700 pregnancies in the developing world[2] and about 1 in 2000 pregnancies in Europe and other developed countries. Eclampsia is often a serious and life-threatening condition. Compared to pre-eclampsia it carries a much higher risk of death and serious morbidity for the woman and her baby. In the UK, for example, 1 in 50 of the women who have eclampsia die[3].

Worldwide, over half a million women die each year of pregnancy-related causes, and 99% of these deaths occur in the developing world[4]. Put another way, women in industrialized countries have an average lifetime risk (calculated as the average number of pregnancies multiplied by the risk associated with each pregnancy) of dying from pregnancy-related causes of between 1 in 4000 and 1 in 10,000, whereas women in low income countries have a risk that is between 1 in 15 and 1 in 50. In poor countries, maternal mortality is 100–200 times higher than in Europe and North America. There is no other public health statistic for which the disparity between rich and poor countries is so wide.

Although rare, eclampsia probably accounts for 50,000 maternal deaths a year[5]. In areas where maternal mortality is very high, infection and haemorrhage are the main causes of death[6], but as deaths from these causes become less common, those associated with pre-eclampsia and eclampsia assume greater importance. Where overall maternal mortality is high, most deaths are associated with eclampsia[5]. In places where mortality is low, a greater proportion of deaths are related to pre-eclampsia. There are few reliable data on the maternal morbidity associated with pre-eclampsia and eclampsia, but it is likely that this is also substantial. In the UK, for example, pre-eclampsia accounts for an estimated one-fifth of antenatal admissions[7], two-thirds of referrals to day care assessment units[8], and a quarter of obstetric admissions to intensive care units[9]. Although maternal mortality in the UK is low, pre-eclampsia/eclampsia accounts for 10–15% of direct obstetric deaths[10,11] as it does in many developing countries[5]. Reducing the morbidity and mortality associated with these conditions is an important priority.

This chapter briefly discusses the classification and pathophysiology of pre-eclampsia and the hypertensive disorders of pregnancy. It then presents the evidence from systematic reviews and randomized trials of the effects of interventions to prevent and treat pre-eclampsia and its complications.

Classification of the hypertensive disorders of pregnancy

Eclampsia and pre-eclampsia are part of a spectrum of conditions associated with raised blood pressure during pregnancy, known as the hypertensive disorders of pregnancy. Attempts to classify these disorders have, in the past, been confusing and sometimes misleading. More recently their classification has been rationalized and simplified to reflect the different situations encountered in clinical practice[12]. Raised blood pressure during pregnancy is generally defined as systolic pressure ≥140 mmHg and/or diastolic pressure ≥90 mmHg, and proteinuria as >300 mg/24 h or ≥30 mg/mmol in a single specimen. There is agreement that the terms pregnancy-induced hypertension, or gestational hypertension, refer to raised blood pressure occurring for the first time in the second half of pregnancy, but without proteinuria (<300 mg/24 h). The term pre-eclampsia is reserved for the new occurrence of hypertension and proteinuria in the second half of pregnancy. The diagnosis of pre-eclampsia is strengthened if there is further indication of multisystem involvement, such as raised serum creatinine or liver enzymes, lowered platelets, or neurological symptoms (hyperreflexia, severe frontal headache, or visual disturbance). Eclampsia is the occurrence of convulsions superimposed on pre-eclampsia. Chronic hypertension is known hypertension before pregnancy. Pre-eclampsia superimposed on chronic hypertension is when a women with chronic hypertension develops new signs or symptoms of pre-eclampsia in the second half of pregnancy.

Women with pregnancy-induced hypertension generally have a good outcome. The risk to them and their baby increases only if they progress to pre-eclampsia, or have very high blood pressure.

Pathophysiology of pre-eclampsia

Although the exact mechanisms which lead to pre-eclampsia are not clear, several factors are known to play a part in determining who will develop this disease. Some women have predisposing factors. These include family history, age and parity. Current thinking is that the primary pathophysiology in pre-eclampsia is placental[13,14]. Pre-eclampsia occurs in women who have an abdominal pregnancy and in those with a hydatidiform mole, indicating that uterine and fetal factors are not essential. In addition, it is more common amongst women who have conditions associated with a large placenta (such as multiple pregnancies and hydrops fetalis), and in women who have microvascular disease (such as diabetes, hypertension and collagen vascular disease). In pre-eclampsia, trophoblastic implantation is abnormal, with reduced placental perfusion. As normal implantation is complete by around 20 weeks, this deficient implantation occurs weeks or months before the disease becomes clinically apparent.

The secondary pathology in pre-eclampsia appears to be endothelial cell injury. The proposed model is that reduced blood supply to the placenta results in production of unknown factors which are released into the maternal circulation and act on endothelial cells, leading to endothelial dysfunction[1]. This results in vasospasm, with consequent reduction in plasma volume, and activation of the coagulation cascade. These changes antedate other clinical findings[1]. Recently, there has been interest in oxidative stress as the possible mechanism for this endothelial dysfunction[1,15].

Interventions to prevent and treat pre-eclampsia and hypertension during pregnancy

The evidence presented here is primarily derived from systematic reviews published on The Cochrane Library[16]. These reviews have a standard and extensive search strategy and methodology, which is described in detail in each of the reviews. Where reviews are not available, evidence is summarized from randomized trials identified by searching the Cochrane Central Controlled Trials Register within The Cochrane Library[16].

Prevention of pre-eclampsia

Diet and exercise

For decades, women have been advised to make a range of changes to their diet and lifestyle, in the expectation that it might reduce their risk of developing pre-eclampsia. Many of these are now obsolete. There is no reliable evidence that any are effective. Interventions that have been evaluated in randomized trials include aerobic exercise[17,18], protein restriction[19], protein supplementation[20,21], increasing or decreasing salt intake[22], magnesium supplementation[23] and zinc supplementation[24]. All the studies in these reviews were small and, even taken together, provide insufficient evidence to provide a reliable basis for clinical decisions. Therefore, in the absence of good evidence of either benefit or harm, women's diet and lifestyle during pregnancy should be determined by their own personal preferences.

Two further forms of supplementation have been evaluated in trials: sources of prostaglandin precursors such as fish oil, and calcium. Fish oil contains long chain fatty acids, which have antiplatelet and antithrombotic effects thought to be beneficial in prevention of pre-eclampsia. Observational studies suggested the possibility of a prophylactic effect of fish oil and prompted more rigorous randomized trials. Other sources of fatty acids, such as oil of evening primrose, have also been evaluated in randomized trials. Over 2000 women have now been randomized into these studies[25]. Taken together, the confidence intervals suggest that the true effect could be anything between a 40% reduction

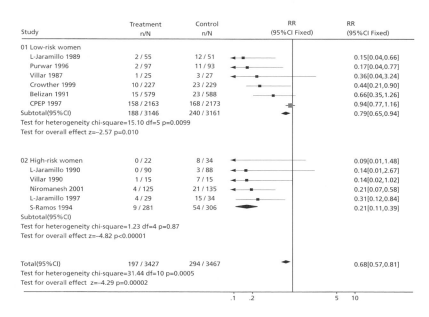

Study	Treatment n/N	Control n/N	RR (95%CI Fixed)	RR (95%CI Fixed)
01 Low-risk women				
L-Jaramillo 1989	2 / 55	12 / 51		0.15[0.04,0.66]
Purwar 1996	2 / 97	11 / 93		0.17[0.04,0.77]
Villar 1987	1 / 25	3 / 27		0.36[0.04,3.24]
Crowther 1999	10 / 227	23 / 229		0.44[0.21,0.90]
Belizan 1991	15 / 579	23 / 588		0.66[0.35,1.26]
CPEP 1997	158 / 2163	168 / 2173		0.94[0.77,1.16]
Subtotal(95%CI)	188 / 3146	240 / 3161		0.79[0.65,0.94]
Test for heterogeneity chi-square=15.10 df=5 p=0.0099				
Test for overall effect z=−2.57 p=0.010				
02 High-risk women	0 / 22	8 / 34		0.09[0.01,1.48]
L-Jaramillo 1990	0 / 90	3 / 88		0.14[0.01,2.67]
Villar 1990	1 / 15	7 / 15		0.14[0.02,1.02]
Niromanesh 2001	4 / 125	21 / 135		0.21[0.07,0.58]
L-Jaramillo 1997	4 / 29	15 / 34		0.31[0.12,0.84]
S-Ramos 1994	9 / 281	54 / 306		0.21[0.11,0.39]
Subtotal(95%CI)				
Test for heterogeneity chi-square=1.23 df=4 p=0.87				
Test for overall effect z=−4.82 p<0.00001				
Total(95%CI)	197 / 3427	294 / 3467		0.68[0.57,0.81]
Test for heterogeneity chi-square=31.44 df=10 p=0.0005				
Test for overall effect z=−4.29 p=0.00002				

Fig. 1 Calcium supplementation *versus* none/placebo: effect on pre-eclampsia (subgroups by maternal risk).

in the risk of pre-eclampsia associated with these oils and a 28% increase [relative risk (RR) 0.87, 95% CI 0.59, 1.28].

The hypothesis that dietary calcium might be related to the risk of pre-eclampsia was also derived from observational studies. There are now 11 trials (6894 women) in the systematic review. Women in these trials received at least 1 g calcium/day[26]. Overall, there is a 30% reduction in the risk of pre-eclampsia (Fig. 1). The effect seems to be greatest for women who were high risk at trial entry (five trials, 587 women; RR 0.21, 95% CI 0.11–0.39), and for those with a previous low calcium intake (six trials, 1842 women; RR 0.32, 95% CI 0.21–0.49)[26]. This reduction in the risk of pre-eclampsia was not reflected in any overall effect on stillbirths or neonatal deaths (nine trials, 6763 women; RR 1.04, 95% CI 0.65, 1.66). A further multicentre trial of women with low dietary calcium was completed in 2003, results are awaited.

Aspirin and other antiplatelet agents
Pre-eclampsia is associated with deficient intravascular production of prostacyclin, a vasodilator, and excessive production of thromboxane, a platelet-derived vasoconstrictor and stimulant of platelet aggregation. These observations led to the hypotheses that antiplatelet agents, and low dose aspirin in particular, might be effective for prevention of pre-eclampsia. There are now 51 trials (36,500 women) in the systematic review[27]. Most women in these trials received low dose (<75 mg)

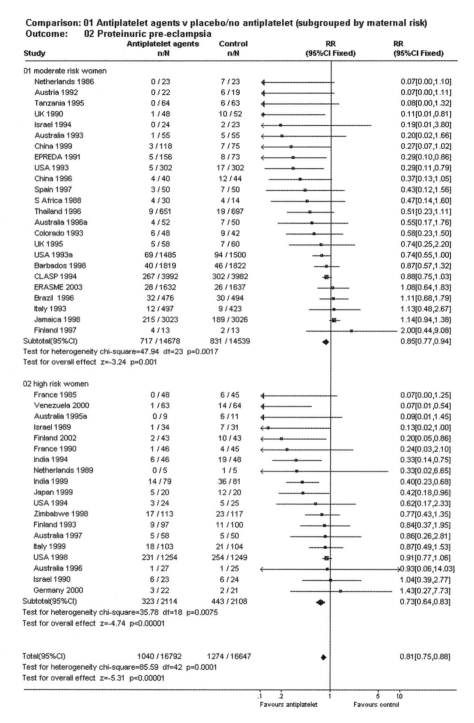

Comparison: 01 Antiplatelet agents v placebo/no antiplatelet (subgrouped by maternal risk)
Outcome: 02 Proteinuric pre-eclampsia

Study	Antiplatelet agents n/N	Control n/N	RR (95%CI Fixed)	RR (95%CI Fixed)
01 moderate risk women				
Netherlands 1986	0 / 23	7 / 23		0.07[0.00,1.10]
Austria 1992	0 / 22	6 / 19		0.07[0.00,1.11]
Tanzania 1995	0 / 64	6 / 63		0.08[0.00,1.32]
UK 1990	1 / 48	10 / 52		0.11[0.01,0.81]
Israel 1994	0 / 24	2 / 23		0.19[0.01,3.80]
Australia 1993	1 / 55	5 / 55		0.20[0.02,1.66]
China 1999	3 / 118	7 / 75		0.27[0.07,1.02]
EPREDA 1991	5 / 156	8 / 73		0.29[0.10,0.86]
USA 1993	5 / 302	17 / 302		0.29[0.11,0.79]
China 1996	4 / 40	12 / 44		0.37[0.13,1.05]
Spain 1997	3 / 50	7 / 50		0.43[0.12,1.56]
S Africa 1988	4 / 30	4 / 14		0.47[0.14,1.60]
Thailand 1996	9 / 651	19 / 697		0.51[0.23,1.11]
Australia 1996a	4 / 52	7 / 50		0.55[0.17,1.76]
Colorado 1993	6 / 48	9 / 42		0.58[0.23,1.50]
UK 1995	5 / 58	7 / 60		0.74[0.25,2.20]
USA 1993a	69 / 1485	94 / 1500		0.74[0.55,1.00]
Barbados 1998	40 / 1819	46 / 1822		0.87[0.57,1.32]
CLASP 1994	267 / 3992	302 / 3982		0.88[0.75,1.03]
ERASME 2003	28 / 1632	26 / 1637		1.08[0.64,1.83]
Brazil 1996	32 / 476	30 / 494		1.11[0.68,1.79]
Italy 1993	12 / 497	9 / 423		1.13[0.48,2.67]
Jamaica 1998	215 / 3023	189 / 3026		1.14[0.94,1.38]
Finland 1997	4 / 13	2 / 13		2.00[0.44,9.08]
Subtotal(95%CI)	717 / 14678	831 / 14539		0.85[0.77,0.94]
Test for heterogeneity chi-square=47.94 df=23 p=0.0017				
Test for overall effect z=-3.24 p=0.001				
02 high risk women				
France 1985	0 / 48	6 / 45		0.07[0.00,1.25]
Venezuela 2000	1 / 63	14 / 64		0.07[0.01,0.54]
Australia 1995a	0 / 9	6 / 11		0.09[0.01,1.45]
Israel 1989	1 / 34	7 / 31		0.13[0.02,1.00]
Finland 2002	2 / 43	10 / 43		0.20[0.05,0.86]
France 1990	1 / 46	4 / 45		0.24[0.03,2.10]
India 1994	6 / 46	19 / 48		0.33[0.14,0.75]
Netherlands 1989	0 / 5	1 / 5		0.33[0.02,6.65]
India 1999	14 / 79	36 / 81		0.40[0.23,0.68]
Japan 1999	5 / 20	12 / 20		0.42[0.18,0.96]
USA 1994	3 / 24	5 / 25		0.62[0.17,2.33]
Zimbabwe 1998	17 / 113	23 / 117		0.77[0.43,1.35]
Finland 1993	9 / 97	11 / 100		0.84[0.37,1.95]
Australia 1997	5 / 58	5 / 50		0.86[0.26,2.81]
Italy 1999	18 / 103	21 / 104		0.87[0.49,1.53]
USA 1998	231 / 1254	254 / 1249		0.91[0.77,1.06]
Australia 1996	1 / 27	1 / 25		0.93[0.06,14.03]
Israel 1990	6 / 23	6 / 24		1.04[0.39,2.77]
Germany 2000	3 / 22	2 / 21		1.43[0.27,7.73]
Subtotal(95%CI)	323 / 2114	443 / 2108		0.73[0.64,0.83]
Test for heterogeneity chi-square=35.78 df=18 p=0.0075				
Test for overall effect z=-4.74 p<0.00001				
Total(95%CI)	1040 / 16792	1274 / 16647		0.81[0.75,0.88]
Test for heterogeneity chi-square=85.59 df=42 p=0.0001				
Test for overall effect z=-5.31 p<0.00001				

.1   .2   1   5   10
Favours antiplatelet   Favours control

Fig. 2   Antiplatelet agents *versus* placebo or no antiplatelet agent: effect on pre-eclampsia (subgroups by maternal risk).

aspirin. Antiplatelet agents are associated with a 19% reduction in the risk of pre-eclampsia [43 trials, 33,439 women; RR 0.81, 95% CI 0.75, 0.88; number needed to treat (NNT) 69, 95% CI 51, 109] (Fig. 2). This reduction is consistent, regardless of risk status or gestation at trial entry. Other benefits associated with antiplatelet agents were: a small (7%) reduction in the risk of delivery before 37 completed weeks (28 trials, 31,845 women; RR 0.93, 95% CI 0.89, 0.98), a 16% reduction in fetal or neonatal deaths (38 trials, 34,010 women; RR 0.84, 95% CI 0.74, 0.96) and an 8% reduction in the risk of a small for gestational age baby (32 trials, 24,310 women; RR 0.92, 95% CI 0.85, 1.00). Low dose aspirin also appears to be reasonably safe.

Low dose aspirin does help prevent pre-eclampsia, and some of its complications. These results should be discussed with women, particularly those at high risk of developing pre-eclampsia. In countries with a high incidence of pre-eclampsia, recommending more widespread use may be worthwhile.

Antioxidant vitamins

One small trial has evaluated high doses of vitamins C and E as antioxidant agents for prevention of pre-eclampsia[28]. The results are promising, but require confirmation in larger studies before being recommended for clinical practice. Several such studies are currently planned or recruiting.

Treatment of mild or moderate hypertension

Mild or moderate hypertension carries little risk to the mother, unless there is superimposed severe hypertension or pre-eclampsia. For this reason, the aim of treatment for mild to moderate hypertension during pregnancy has been to defer or prevent the progression to severe hypertension or pre-eclampsia. Rest in bed and a variety of medications have been used.

Bed rest

Women with high blood pressure during pregnancy have often been advised to rest in bed, either at home or in hospital. Confinement to bed either at home or in hospital may result in financial or social costs for the woman and her family. Admission to hospital may be stressful and has, in addition, major cost implications for the health services. These interventions would only be justified if there were clear health benefits. Three small trials (408 women) have compared hospital admission with care at home for hypertension alone[29]. Two trials (145 women) have compared bed rest in hospital with normal ambulation for women with pre-eclampsia. Even taken together, these trials are too small for any reliable conclusions[30].

Antihypertensive agents

Antihypertensive agents are used to lower blood pressure during pregnancy, in the belief that these delay progression to more severe disease, and so improve outcome. Twenty-four trials (2815 women) have compared an antihypertensive drug with placebo/no antihypertensive drug for women with mild–moderate hypertension during pregnancy[31]. Unsurprisingly, antihypertensive drugs reduce by half the risk of developing severe hypertension (17 trials, 2155 women; RR 0.52, 95% CI 0.41, 0.64), but with little evidence of a difference in the risk of pre-eclampsia (19 trials, 2402 women; RR 0.99, 95% CI 0.84, 1.18) (Fig. 3). Similarly, there is no clear effect on the risk of the baby dying (23 trials, 2727 women; RR 0.71, 95% CI 0.46, 1.09), being born too early (12 trials, 1738 women; RR 0.98, 95% CI 0.85, 1.13), or being small for gestational age (17 trials, 2159 women; RR 1.13, 95% CI 0.91, 1.42).

Possible adverse effects are not well reported in these trials. There is a trend towards an increase in small for gestational age babies, largely confined to the beta blocker group of drugs[31]. Meta-regression within a systematic review has suggested that lowering blood pressure may increase the risk of a small for gestational age baby[32]. There are few data to provide reassurance on long-term follow-up for either the mother or baby.

It remains unclear whether antihypertensive drug therapy for mild–moderate hypertension during pregnancy is worthwhile. Whether the reduction in the risk of severe hypertension is considered sufficient to warrant treatment is a decision that should be made by women in consultation with their obstetrician. If an antihypertensive is used, there is little good evidence that one antihypertensive is clearly better than another. The choice should therefore depend on the previous experience of the clinician and the woman's preference.

Treatment of severe hypertension/pre-eclampsia

Antihypertensive drugs

Although treatment of hypertension does not strike at the basic disorder, it may still benefit the mother and fetus. An important objective in the care of a woman with severe hypertension, with or without proteinuria, is to reduce blood pressure in order to avoid hypertensive encephalopathy and cerebral haemorrhage. For this reason, the aim in treating severely hypertensive women is to keep the blood pressure below dangerous levels (< 170/110 mmHg).

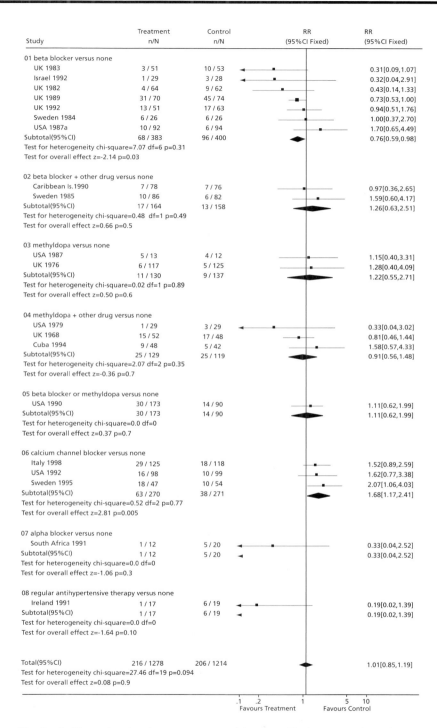

Fig. 3 Antihypertensive drugs *versus* none/placebo: effect on pre-eclampsia (subgroups by type of drug).

Twenty trials (1637 women) have compared one antihypertensive agent with another for severe hypertension[33]. Most of these studies were small. There are 10 comparisons in the review, five of which compared hydralazine with another drug. Other agents included were nifedipine, labetolol, methyldopa, diazoxide, prostacyclin, ketanserin, urapidil, magnesium sulphate, prazosin and nimodipine.

There is no good evidence that one antihypertensive is better than any of the others for reducing blood pressure. Until better evidence is available, the best choice of drug for an individual woman probably depends on the experience and familiarity of her clinician with a particular drug, and on what is known about adverse maternal and fetal side-effects. Diazoxide is probably best avoided, however, as although the numbers are small it does seem to be associated with an increased risk of very low blood pressure and of caesarean section when compared to labetolol. Also, ketanserin is less effective in reducing blood pressure than hydralazine.

Plasma volume expansion

Women with severe pre-eclampsia often have a restricted circulating plasma volume. This has led to the recommendation that plasma volume should be expanded with either colloid or crystalloid solutions, in an effort to improve maternal systemic and uteroplacental circulation. However, intravascular volume expansion carries a serious risk of volume overload, which may lead to pulmonary or cerebral oedema. Also, large volume expansion often requires invasive monitoring of intravascular pressure, procedures carrying risks of their own.

Three small trials (61 women) have compared a colloid solution with placebo or no infusion. These studies were too small for reliable conclusions, but suggest plasma volume expansion is not beneficial[34]. Systematic reviews of volume expansion for critically ill non-pregnant people found a higher mortality than either not using any plasma expander or expansion with a crystalloid[35,36]. Although none of these studies included pregnant women, it would seem prudent to avoid colloid solutions until data from randomized trials involving women with pre-eclampsia become available.

Timing of delivery

For women who have severe pre-eclampsia before 34 weeks, the decision about the best time to deliver the baby is often difficult. The hazards to the baby of being born too early need to be balanced against the risks to both the woman and the baby if the pregnancy is continued for too long. Two trials (133 women) have compared a policy of early elective delivery by induction of labour or by caesarean section, with a policy of delayed delivery. There are insufficient data for any reliable recommendation about which policy of care should be used for women with severe early onset pre-eclampsia.

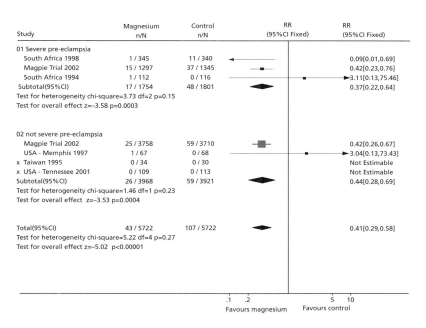

Study	Magnesium n/N	Control n/N	RR (95%CI Fixed)	RR (95%CI Fixed)
01 Severe pre-eclampsia				
South Africa 1998	1 / 345	11 / 340		0.09[0.01,0.69]
Magpie Trial 2002	15 / 1297	37 / 1345		0.42[0.23,0.76]
South Africa 1994	1 / 112	0 / 116		3.11[0.13,75.46]
Subtotal(95%CI)	17 / 1754	48 / 1801		0.37[0.22,0.64]
Test for heterogeneity chi-square=3.73 df=2 p=0.15				
Test for overall effect z=−3.58 p=0.0003				
02 not severe pre-eclampsia				
Magpie Trial 2002	25 / 3758	59 / 3710		0.42[0.26,0.67]
USA - Memphis 1997	1 / 67	0 / 68		3.04[0.13,73.43]
x Taiwan 1995	0 / 34	0 / 30		Not Estimable
x USA - Tennessee 2001	0 / 109	0 / 113		Not Estimable
Subtotal(95%CI)	26 / 3968	59 / 3921		0.44[0.28,0.69]
Test for heterogeneity chi-square=1.46 df=1 p=0.23				
Test for overall effect z=−3.53 p=0.0004				
Total(95%CI)	43 / 5722	107 / 5722		0.41[0.29,0.58]
Test for heterogeneity chi-square=5.22 df=4 p=0.27				
Test for overall effect z=−5.02 p<0.00001				

.1   .2   5   10
Favours magnesium   Favours control

Fig. 4 Magnesium sulphate *versus* none/placebo: effect on eclampsia (subgroups by severity of pre-eclampsia).

Prevention and treatment of eclampsia

Anticonvulsant drugs are widely used in the management of eclampsia, as well as in severe hypertensive disease and pre-eclampsia, in an attempt to prevent the occurrence of eclamptic seizures. Magnesium sulphate has recently emerged as the anticonvulsant of choice for eclampsia.

Preventing the onset of eclampsia

The main question about magnesium sulphate as a prophylactic anticonvulsant for women with pre-eclampsia is whether overall it does more good than harm. Six trials (11,444 women) have compared magnesium sulphate with placebo or no anticonvulsant[37]. Most women in these studies had moderate–severe pre-eclampsia. The magnesium sulphate regimen was usually 4 g as a slow intravenous bolus, followed by either an intravenous infusion of 1 g/h, or by intramuscular injections of 10 g and then 5 g every 4 h. The total duration of therapy was usually 24 h, with clinical monitoring alone.

There was more than a halving in the risk of eclampsia associated with the use of magnesium sulphate, rather than placebo or no anticonvulsant (RR 0.41, 95% CI 0.29, 0.58; NNT 100, 95% CI 50–100). This reduction is consistent regardless of severity of pre-eclampsia (Fig. 4) and irrespective of gestation or whether the women were antepartum at trial entry. The risk of maternal death was also reduced for women allocated magnesium sulphate, although this did not achieve statistical significance (two trials, 10,795 women; RR 0.54, 95% CI 0.26, 1.10). There was no clear evidence of any overall difference in maternal morbidity between the two groups.

For women randomized before delivery, the risk of placental abruption was reduced for those allocated magnesium sulphate rather than placebo (RR 0.64, 95% CI 0.50–0.83). Women allocated magnesium sulphate also had a small (5%) increase in the risk of caesarean section (six trials, 10,108 women; RR 1.05, 95% CI 1.01, 1.10). There was no evidence of a clinically important effect on the risk of induction of labour, postpartum haemorrhage or manual removal of placenta. There was no overall difference in the risk of stillbirth or neonatal death (three trials, 9961 women; RR 1.04, 95% CI 0.93, 1.15) or in the risk of the baby dying or being in a special care baby unit for >7 days (RR 1.01, 95% CI 0.95–1.08). There was no clear difference in neonatal morbidity between the two groups. Follow-up after discharge from hospital is being conducted for one large trial[38], but data are not yet available.

Toxicity was uncommon with magnesium sulphate. There was no clear difference in the risk of absent or reduced tendon reflexes. Although respiratory depression was rare (52/5344 *versus* 26/5333), the risk was higher for women allocated magnesium sulphate (RR 1.98, 95% CI 1.24–3.15; NNH 206, 95% CI 100–1000). A quarter of women who received magnesium sulphate had side-effects, compared to 5% of those given placebo. By far the most common side-effect was flushing.

Trials have also compared magnesium sulphate with phenytoin (two trials, 2241 women) with nimodipine (one trial, 1750 women), and with diazepam (two trials, 66 women). These studies all support magnesium sulphate as the anticonvulsant of choice for women with pre-eclampsia. One trial has compared magnesium chloride with methyldopa (31 women).

Magnesium sulphate should be considered for women with severe pre-eclampsia, and for others about whom there is concern about the risk of eclampsia.

Controlling the acute convulsion and preventing recurrence of eclampsia

When a woman has an eclamptic convulsion, the immediate question is how best to control the acute fit. Once the first convulsion has subsided, the next question is how best to reduce the risk of her having another. In the past, the choice of anticonvulsant was controversial, but magnesium sulphate is now well established as the drug of choice.

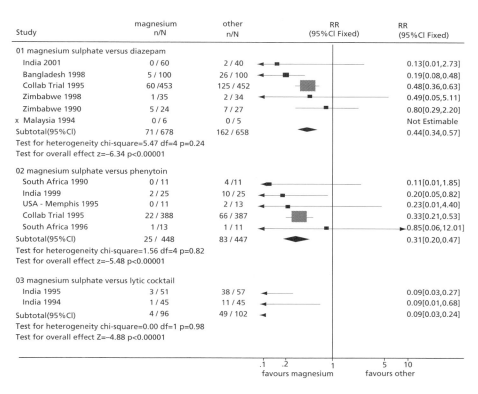

Fig. 5 Magnesium sulphate *versus* other anticonvulsants: effect on recurrence of convulsio

Magnesium sulphate has been compared with diazepam, with pheny-toin, and with lytic cocktail in randomized trials. Six trials (1336 women) have compared magnesium sulphate with diazepam[39]. Magnesium sulphate was associated with a reduction in the risk of maternal death, when compared to diazepam, although the confidence intervals are wide (RR 0.59, 95% CI 0.37, 0.94). There is also a substantial reduction in the risk of recurrence of convulsions associated with magnesium sulphate (RR 0.44, 95% CI 0.34–0.57) (Fig. 5). On average, for every seven women treated with magnesium sulphate rather than diazepam, one recurrence of convulsions will be prevented (95% CI 6–10 women). There was no clear evidence of a difference in any other measure of maternal morbidity.

For the baby, there was no clear difference between the treatment regimens in the risk of perinatal death for babies randomized whilst *in utero* (RR 1.04, 95% CI 0.80, 1.36). The only clear differences associated with the use of magnesium sulphate, rather than diazepam, were a reduction in the risk of an Apgar score <7 at 5 min (RR 0.72, 95% CI 0.55–0.94), and in length of stay in a special care baby unit >7 days (RR 0.66, 95% CI 0.46–0.95).

Six trials (897 women) have compared magnesium sulphate with phenytoin[40]. Magnesium sulphate was associated with a 70% reduction in the relative risk of recurrent convulsions, compared to phenytoin (RR 0.31, 95% CI 0.20–0.47) (Fig. 5). On average, for every eight women treated with magnesium sulphate rather than phenytoin, one recurrence of convulsions will be prevented (95% CI 6–13 women). The trend in maternal mortality also favoured magnesium sulphate, but the difference did not achieve statistical significance (RR 0.50, 95% CI 0.24–1.05). In addition, the use of magnesium sulphate, rather than phenytoin, was associated with a reduction in the risk of pneumonia (RR 0.44, 95% CI 0.24–0.79), the need for ventilation (RR 0.66, 95% CI 0.49–0.90) and admission to an intensive care unit (RR 0.67, 95% CI 0.50–0.89).

For the baby, there was no clear difference in the risk of perinatal death between the two regimens (RR 0.85, 95% CI 0.67, 1.09). Babies whose mothers were allocated magnesium sulphate, rather than phenytoin, had fewer admissions to a special care baby unit (RR 0.73, 95% CI 0.58–0.91) and fewer died or were in SCBU for >7 days (RR 0.77, 95% CI 0.63–0.95).

Two trials (199 women) compared magnesium sulphate with lytic cocktail[41], usually a mixture of chlorpromazine, promethazine and pethidine. Magnesium sulphate was substantially better at preventing further fits than lytic cocktail (RR 0.09, 95% CI 0.03, 0.24). There was also a non-significant trend to fewer maternal deaths with magnesium sulphate rather than lytic cocktail (RR 0.25, 95% CI 0.04–1.43), and fewer baby deaths (for stillbirth RR 0.55, 95% CI 0.26–1.16; for neonatal death RR 0.39, 95% CI 0.14–1.06).

Magnesium sulphate is the drug of choice for women with eclampsia. In these trials, women allocated magnesium sulphate had magnesium sulphate for treatment of the acute fit, for maintenance therapy and for control of any recurrent fits. The treatment regimens were similar to those discussed above for pre-eclampsia. It has been argued that diazepam should be used for control of the acute fit[42], but this view is not supported by evidence[43].

Conclusions

A wide range of interventions has been suggested for the prevention and treatment of pre-eclampsia. Many thousands of women have now been entered into randomized trials evaluating some of these interventions, and this evidence provides the basis for a more rational approach to some aspects of care. Many important unanswered questions remain, however. Further improvement in the care of women with pre-eclampsia will come from implementing the existing evidence, and from conducting further large trials to evaluate interventions not yet tested in large trials.

References

1 Roberts JM, Redman CW. Pre-eclampsia: more than pregnancy-induced hypertension. *Lancet* 1993; **341**: 1447–51
2 Bergstrom S, Povey G, Songane F, Ching C. Seasonal incidence of eclampsia and its relationship to meteorological data in Mozambique. *J Perinat Med* 1992; **20**: 153–8
3 Douglas KA, Redman CW. Eclampsia in the United Kingdom. *BMJ* 1994; **309**: 1395–400
4 Mahler H. The safe motherhood initiative: a call to action. *Lancet* 1987; **1**: 668–70
5 Duley L. Maternal mortality associated with hypertensive disorders of pregnancy in Africa, Asia, Latin America and the Caribbean. *Br J Obstet Gynaecol* 1992; **99**: 547–53
6 Loudon I. *Death in Childbed: An International Study of Maternal Care and Maternal Mortality 1800–1950*. Oxford: Clarendon Press, 1992
7 Rosenberg K, Twaddle S. Screening and surveillance of pregnancy hypertension—an economic approach to the use of daycare. *Baillière's Clin Obstet Gynaecol* 1990; **4**: 89–107
8 Anthony J. Improving antenatal care: the role of an antenatal assessment unit. *Health Trends* 1992; **24**: 123–5
9 Bouvier-Colle MH, Salanave B, Ancel PY *et al*. Obstetric patients treated in intensive care units and maternal mortality. Regional Teams for the Survey. *Eur J Obstet Gynecol Reprod Biol* 1996; **65**: 121–5
10 Department of Health, Welsh Office, Scottish Home and Health Department, Northern Ireland, Department of Health and Social Services. *Report on Confidential Enquiries into Maternal Deaths in the United Kingdom 1991–1993*. London: HMSO, 1996
11 Department of Health, Welsh Office, Scottish Office Department of Health, Department of Health and Social Services NI. *Why Mothers Die: Report on Confidential Enquiries into Maternal Deaths in the United Kingdom, 1994–1996: Executive Summary and Key Recommendations*. London: TSO, c1998, 1998
12 Brown MA, Lindheimer MD, de Swiet M, Van Assche A, Moutquin JM. The classification and diagnosis of the hypertensive disorders of pregnancy: statement from the International Society for the Study of Hypertension in Pregnancy (ISSHP). *Hypertens Pregnancy* 2001; **20**: IX–XIV
13 Roberts JM, Cooper DW. Pathogenesis and genetics of pre-eclampsia. *Lancet* 2001; **357**: 53–6
14 Roberts JM, Lain KY. Recent insights into the pathogenesis of pre-eclampsia. *Placenta* 2002; **23**: 359–72
15 Hubel CA. Oxidative stress in the pathogenesis of preeclampsia. *Proc Soc Exp Biol Med* 1999; **222**: 222–35
16 *The Cochrane Library*. Oxford: Update Software
17 Kramer MS. Aerobic exercise for women during pregnancy. In: *The Cochrane Library, Issue 1, 2003*. Oxford: Update Software
18 Kramer MS. Regular aerobic exercise during pregnancy. In: *The Cochrane Library, Issue 1, 2003*. Oxford: Update Software
19 Kramer MS. Energy/protein restriction for high weight-for-height or weight gain during pregnancy. In: *The Cochrane Library, Issue 1, 2003*. Oxford: Update Software
20 Kramer MS. Isocaloric balanced protein supplementation in pregnancy. In: *The Cochrane Library, Issue 1, 2003*. Oxford: Update Software
21 Kramer MS. Balanced protein/energy supplementation in pregnancy. In: *The Cochrane Library, Issue 1, 2003*. Oxford: Update Software
22 Duley L, Henderson-Smart D. Reduced salt intake compared to normal dietary salt, or high intake, in pregnancy. In: *The Cochrane Library, Issue 1, 2003*. Oxford: Update Software
23 Makrides M, Crowther CA. Magnesium supplementation in pregnancy. In: *The Cochrane Library, Issue 1, 2003*. Oxford: Update Software

24 Mahomed K. Zinc supplementation in pregnancy. In: *The Cochrane Library, Issue 1*, 2003. Oxford: Update Software

25 Makrides M, Duley L, Olsen SF. Fish oil, and other prostaglandin precursor, supplementation during pregnancy to improve outcomes in pre-eclampsia, preterm birth, low birth weight and small for gestational age. In: *The Cochrane Library, Issue 1*, 2003. Oxford: Update Software

26 Atallah AN, Hofmeyr GJ, Duley L. Calcium supplementation during pregnancy for preventing hypertensive disorders and related problems (Cochrane Review). In: *The Cochrane Library, Issue 1*, 2003. Oxford: Update Software

27 Knight M, Duley L, Henderson-Smart DJ, King JF. Antiplatelet agents for preventing and treating pre-eclampsia. In: *The Cochrane Library, Issue 1*, 2003. Oxford: Update Software

28 Chappell LC, Seed PT, Briley AL *et al*. Effect of antioxidants on the occurrence of pre-eclampsia in women at increased risk: a randomised trial. *Lancet* 1999; **354**: 810–6

29 Duley L. Hospitalisation for non-proteinuric pregnancy hypertension. In: *The Cochrane Library, Issue 2*, 1995. Oxford: Update Software

30 Duley L. Strict bed rest for proteinuric hypertension in pregnancy. In: *The Cochrane Library, Issue 2*, 1995. Oxford: Update Software

31 Abalos E, Duley L, Steyn DW, Henderson-Smart DJ. Antihypertensive drug therapy for mild to moderate hypertension during pregnancy. In: *The Cochrane Library, Issue 1*, 2003. Oxford: Update Software

32 von Dadelszen P, Ornstein MP, Bull SB, Logan AG, Koren G, Magee LA. Fall in mean arterial pressure and fetal growth restriction in pregnancy hypertension: a meta-analysis. *Lancet* 2000; **355**: 87–92

33 Duley L, Henderson-Smart DJ. Drugs for rapid treatment of very high blood pressure during pregnancy. In: *The Cochrane Library, Issue 1*, 2003. Oxford: Update Software

34 Duley L, Williams J, Henderson-Smart DJ. Plasma volume expansion for treatment of women with pre-eclampsia. In: *The Cochrane Library, Issue 1*, 2003. Oxford: Update Software

35 Alderson P, Bunn F, Lefebvre C *et al*. Human albumin solution for resuscitation and volume expansion in critically ill patients. In: *The Cochrane Library, Issue 1*, 2003. Oxford: Update Software

36 Alderson P, Schierhout G, Roberts I, Bunn F. Colloids versus crystalloids for fluid resuscitation in critically ill patients. In: *The Cochrane Library, Issue 1*, 2003. Oxford: Update Software

37 Duley L, Gulmezoglu AM, Henderson-Smart DJ. Magnesium sulphate and other anticonvulsants for women with pre-eclampsia. In: *The Cochrane Library, Issue 1*, 2003. Oxford: Update Software

38 Magpie Trial Collaborative Group. Do women with pre-eclampsia, and their babies, benefit from magnesium sulphate? The Magpie Trial: a randomised placebo-controlled trial. *Lancet* 2002; **359**: 1877–90

39 Duley L, Henderson-Smart D. Magnesium sulphate versus diazepam for eclampsia. In: *The Cochrane Library, Issue 1*, 2003. Oxford: Update Software

40 Duley L, Henderson-Smart D. Magnesium sulphate versus phenytoin for eclampsia. In: *The Cochrane Library, Issue 1*, 2003. Oxford: Update Software

41 Duley L, Gulmezoglu AM. Magnesium sulphate versus lytic cocktail for eclampsia. In: *The Cochrane Library, Issue 1*, 2003. Oxford: Update Software

42 Fox R, Draycott T. Prefer diazepam for initial control of pre-eclamptic fits. *BMJ* 1995; **311**: 1433

43 Duley L. Magnesium sulphate should be used for eclamptic fits. *BMJ* 1996; **312**: 639

Thromboembolism

James Drife

Department of Obstetrics and Gynaecology, University of Leeds, Leeds, UK

Venous thomboembolism (VTE) causes only about 2% of maternal deaths in the developing world but is a leading cause of direct maternal deaths in developed countries. Pregnancy increases the risk of VTE through venous stasis, changes in blood coagulability and damage to vessels. Early diagnosis of VTE depends crucially on awareness of the condition but clinical diagnosis is unreliable in pregnancy and objective testing is essential. Compression or duplex ultrasonography is used to diagnose deep venous thrombosis and a ventilation/perfusion scan for pulmonary embolism. Low molecular weight heparins are safe and effective for treatment and for thromboprophylaxis in pregnancy. All women should undergo risk assessment in early pregnancy or preferably before pregnancy. Identifying risk factors such as obesity, or a past or family history of thromboembolism, allows at-risk women to be offered thromboprophylaxis. Guidelines on thromboprophylaxis have reduced deaths after caesarean section and are now being developed for all women.

Introduction

During pregnancy and the puerperium the risk of thromboembolism is increased compared to the non-pregnant state. In most parts of the world this is overshadowed by other complications of pregnancy which account for a much greater proportion of maternal mortality and morbidity. In developed countries, however, as mortality from other causes has been reduced, thromboembolism has emerged as a leading cause of maternal death.

Thromboembolism occurs mainly in women with other risk factors in addition to pregnancy. Attention is now focused on identifying such women and targeting prophylactic measures, and this will be discussed later in this chapter. Recognition and appropriate management of early disease are also important if morbidity and mortality are to be reduced, and this chapter discusses diagnosis and treatment of thromboembolic disorders as well as their prevention.

Correspondence to:
Prof. James Drife,
Department of Obstetrics
and Gynaecology, Level D,
Clarendon Wing,
Belmont Grove,
Leeds LS2 9NS, UK.
E-mail:
j.o.drife@leeds.ac.uk

British Medical Bulletin 2003; **67**: 177–190
DOI: 10.1093/bmb/ldg010

Incidence

Venous thromboembolic disease has an estimated annual incidence in developed countries of 1 in 1000 people[1]. The figure increases with age from 1 in 100,000 in childhood to nearly 1% in old age[2]. Among non-pregnant young women the incidence is 1 in 20,000 per year (and 1 in 6600 among those using second-generation oral contraceptives)[3]. In pregnancy the incidence is 1 in 1200 pregnancies but it is also related to age[4]: in women under 35 it is about 1 in 1600 pregnancies[3,5]—about 12 times that in non-pregnant young women—but over the age of 35 it is about 1 in 800[4,5].

The mortality is 1–2%[2]. Pregnancy-associated death from thromboembolism occurs once in around 70,000 pregnancies[6]—again, a 12-fold increase compared to the non-pregnant state, where the risk is around one in a million. By comparison, the contraceptive pill increases the risk approximately three-fold[7]. The risks of thrombosis with the pill are better known than those of pregnancy, and it is regrettable that inaccurate perceptions are helping to restrict the pill's availability in countries where it could help to reduce maternal mortality by preventing unwanted pregnancy[8].

Contribution to maternal mortality

Globally, thromboembolism is not among the leading causes of maternal mortality as estimated by the World Health Organization. Most of the world's maternal deaths occur in developing countries, where other causes predominate. In a hospital-based study in rural Ghana, embolism accounted for 2.2% of direct deaths (five out of 156 cases)[9] and in the second report on Confidential Enquiries into Maternal Deaths in South Africa (1999–2001), thromboembolism also caused 2% of direct deaths (48 out of 1462 cases)[10]. In a comparison of hospitals in Zambia and the USA, pulmonary embolism did not figure among the 45 deaths in the Zambian hospital but caused 15% of the 20 deaths in the US hospital[11].

In the USA in 1991–1997 there were 3201 pregnancy-related deaths, with hypertensive disorders accounting for 509, infection for 422, haemorrhage for 401, and thrombotic embolism for 327[12]. Compared to the UK, thromboembolism seems under-represented, bearing in mind the importance of obesity as a risk factor in both countries. The pattern in the USA may be due to suboptimal management of the other conditions (there has been no improvement in maternal mortality in the USA since 1982)[12] or to under-reporting of thromboembolic deaths, many of which occur outside hospital.

In Europe there is a variable picture of under-reporting of direct deaths[13,14] but data from the UK are among the most accurate. In England

and Wales thromboembolism has been one of the major causes of maternal mortality since 1952, when confidential enquiries into maternal deaths began. Table 1 shows that deaths from all the leading causes fell between 1952 and 1984, but the fall in deaths from pulmonary embolism was less than the others.

Since 1973 in England and Wales there has been no reduction in the number of deaths from pulmonary embolism, and from 1991 onwards it has been the leading cause of maternal death in the UK, with 30 deaths in 1991–1993 and 46 in 1994–1996. In 1997–1999 there were 31 deaths, equating to a rate of 14 per million maternities. In addition, however, there were 14 'late' deaths from this cause, so the true rate is probably 50% higher.

In 1997–1999 more than half of the antepartum deaths were in the first trimester, before the woman had booked for antenatal care. Table 2 shows the striking reduction in deaths after caesarean section (despite an increasing national caesarean section rate), which is discussed in the final section of this chapter. Of the 10 deaths after vaginal delivery, most occurred after the woman had been discharged from hospital (Table 3).

Of the 18 deaths after vaginal delivery (including eight late deaths), only one followed instrumental delivery. Most of the women who died

Table 1 Main causes of direct maternal death in England and Wales, 1952–1984

	Abortion	**Pulmonary embolism**	Haemorrhage	Hypertensive disease	All other causes	Total
1952–54	153	**138**	220	246	369	1094
1961–63	139	**129**	92	104	228	692
1970–72	81	**61**	27	47	139	355
1973–75	29	**35**	21	39	111	235
1976–78	19	**45**	26	29	108	227
1979–81	14	**23**	14	36	89	176
1982–84	11	**25**	9	25	68	138

Adapted from CEMD reports[15,16].

Table 2 Deaths from pulmonary embolism (excluding *late* deaths), UK, 1985–99

	Antepartum deaths	Deaths after caesarean section	Deaths after vaginal delivery	Total (including deaths after miscarriage, ectopic and in labour)
1985–87	16	7	6	30
1988–90	10	8	3	24
1991–93	12	13	4	30
1994–96	15	15	10	46
1997–99	13	4[a]	10	31

From 'Why Mothers Die'[6].
[a]Another three deaths followed caesarean section which was carried out after antepartum collapse.

Table 3 Interval between delivery and death from pulmonary embolism, UK, 1997–99

	Days post-partum					Total
	0–7	8–14	15–28	29–42	43–365	
Vaginal delivery	1	2	4	3	8	18
Caesarean section[a]	3	–	–	1	1	5
Total	4	2	4	4	9	23

From 'Why Mothers Die'[6].
[a]Another three deaths followed caesarean section carried out after antepartum collapse.

in 1997–1999 had risk factors in addition to pregnancy and in particular many were overweight.

Pathology

Pathogenesis of thromboembolism

Virchow's triad, described almost 150 years ago[2], consists of venous stasis, changes in the vessel wall and changes in the composition of the blood. Pregnancy affects all three factors. Firstly, progestogen-mediated changes to the blood vessels cause venous stasis, which begins by the end of the first trimester and is greatest at 36 weeks. Compression of the pelvic veins adds to this in later pregnancy and affects particularly the left side: almost 90% of deep venous thrombosis (DVT) is on the left side in pregnancy, compared to 55% in the non-pregnant state. More worryingly, 72% of DVT in pregnancy is ileofemoral (compared to 9% in the non-pregnant) and therefore more likely to embolize[5].

Secondly, the endothelium of the walls of the pelvic veins may be damaged during vaginal delivery or at caesarean section. Thirdly, clotting factors alter in pregnancy. There are increases in factors V and VIII and fibrinogen, acquired resistance to activated protein C (an endogenous anticoagulant) and a reduction in its co-factor, protein S. There are also increases in inhibitors of plasminogen activator, resulting in impaired fibrinolysis[5].

Congenital thrombophilia

Since the first description in 1965 of a family with hereditary thrombosis[2], a number of thrombophilias have been discovered. The most common abnormality underlying venous thromboembolism is factor V Leiden, and the other main thrombophilias include deficiencies of protein C and protein S. Antithrombin III deficiency is the rarest but carries the highest thrombogenic risk[17].

Clinical thrombosis is now recognized to be a multicausal disease resulting from interaction between congenital and acquired risk factors[2,5]. Thrombophilias interact with pregnancy. Among pregnant women with antithrombin deficiency the incidence of thromboembolism has been estimated at 32–44%[5]. With protein C and protein S deficiency the risks of thrombosis in pregnancy have been estimated at 3–10% and 0–6%, respectively.

Consequences of thromboembolism

As well as fatal pulmonary embolism (PE), venous thrombosis results in a disabling post-thrombotic syndrome in at least 20% of patients[2]. Chronic venous hypertension causes limb pain, swelling, hyperpigmentation, dermatitis, ulcers, venous gangrene and lipodermatosclerosis[1]. In one survey of patients 9–144 months (mean 41 months) after DVT, 49% had pain, 26% pigmentation, 21% oedema and 3% ulceration[18]. Post-thrombotic syndrome has a significant impact on quality of life, which worsens with increasing severity of the syndrome[19].

Diagnosis

The diagnosis of thromboembolism depends first and foremost on awareness of the condition. Successive reports from the UK confidential enquiries have included the histories of women whose doctors—in general practice, accident and emergency departments and specialist units—failed to recognize classic symptoms, even when risk factors such as obesity or a family history were present.

Symptoms and signs

With DVT, pain or swelling of the leg (particularly the left leg) are the common presenting complaints. Other features include tenderness, increased temperature, lower abdominal pain or a raised white cell count. Clinical diagnosis is unreliable, however, and less than half the cases suspected clinically are confirmed on objective testing. Even in the non-pregnant woman, individual signs and symptoms are of little value and 'Homan's sign' is of no value. In pregnancy, pitting oedema may be physiological and structured clinical models for diagnosis may not be valid[1,20]. Nevertheless, features such as a history of immobilization, asymmetrical calf swelling (>3 cm difference in calf circumference measured 10 cm below the tibial tuberosity) or swelling of the entire leg are still important in pregnancy[1,21].

PE normally produces symptoms and signs and rarely causes sudden death without warning. Dyspnoea is the main clinical feature, usually associated with chest pain. Other features are faintness or collapse, haemoptysis, focal signs in the chest, raised jugular venous pulse and signs or symptoms of DVT.

The Royal College of Obstetricians and Gynaecologists (RCOG) has produced a detailed guideline on the management of thromboembolic disease in pregnancy and the puerperium[21]. It points out that in pregnancy the vast majority of DVTs are ileofemoral and will therefore require treatment, and advises that when the condition is suspected clinically, anticoagulant treatment should be started until an objective diagnosis is made. It states: 'Any woman with signs and symptoms suggestive of venous thromboembolism should have objective testing carried out expeditiously to avoid the risks, inconvenience and costs of inappropriate anticoagulation. Individual hospitals should have an agreed protocol for the objective diagnosis of suspected venous thromboembolism during pregnancy.'

Screening tests

D-dimers are derivatives of fibrin, produced by plasmin degradation, and several assays are available to measure circulating levels. In the non-pregnant, D-dimer testing is useful because of the high negative predictive value if the blood level is low, and this is also true in pregnancy. D-dimer levels can be elevated in pregnancy, however, particularly if there is also pre-eclampsia, so a positive test is unhelpful.

Definitive investigations

For DVT, the diagnostic gold standard has been contrast venography but this is invasive and ultrasonography is now preferred. Compression ultrasound involves gently pressing the vascular lumen with the ultrasound probe: a fully compressible vein indicates the absence of thrombosis. Duplex ultrasonography involves additionally evaluating the blood flow characteristics with pulsed Doppler: normal flow is phasic with respiration, and absence of this phasic pattern indicates venous outflow obstruction[1].

If ultrasound is negative and there is a low index of clinical suspicion, anticoagulant treatment can be discontinued but if there is a high level of clinical suspicion, anticoagulant treatment should be continued and the ultrasound examination repeated in 1 week. X-ray venography may be considered. If the repeat examination is also negative, treatment may be discontinued then[20,21].

For PE, the cornerstone of diagnosis is the ventilation/perfusion (V/Q) scan, though in many places spiral computed tomography is now the first-line imaging technique in the non-pregnant[22]. When PE is suspected in pregnancy, ultrasound examination for DVT should be carried out[20,21] and a chest X-ray should be done if another diagnosis is considered possible[20]. If these examinations are negative a V/Q scan should be carried out, though a perfusion scan alone may be sufficient. If the V/Q scan reports a low probability of PE, treatment should nevertheless be continued if either the ultrasound investigation is positive or the clinical suspicion is high, in which case further investigation by angiography, magnetic resonance imaging or spiral computed tomography (if postpartum) should be considered.

A pregnant woman who is advised to undergo radiological investigation will be concerned about the risk to her baby. She can be reassured that the radiation dose from either a chest X-ray or venography with abdominal shielding is extremely low[20]. The reports of the UK Confidential Enquiries into Maternal Deaths have repeatedly stressed that chest X-rays are not contraindicated in pregnancy, and the most recent report advises that 'pregnancy is not a reason for withholding plain X-ray films of the abdomen, chest X-rays, some CT scans or MRI from sick women'[6].

Treatment

Patients with suspected thromboembolism should be treated with heparin until the diagnosis has been confirmed or excluded, unless treatment is strongly contraindicated. A thrombophilia screen, full blood count and coagulation screen should be checked before treatment, bearing in mind that pregnancy may affect the thrombophilia screen (for example, protein S levels fall in normal pregnancy).

Initial treatment

Standard initial treatment has been unfractionated heparin, which reduces the risk of extension of thromboembolism compared to oral anticoagulation only. The most common mistake when starting treatment is failure to achieve adequate anticoagulation[23] but achieving the target activated partial thromboplastin time (APTT) may be difficult in late pregnancy, when pregnancy-induced changes produce apparent heparin resistance, and monitoring may require measurement of factor Xa levels. The need for APTT monitoring can be avoided by the use of low molecular weight heparins.

Intravenous unfractionated heparin remains the treatment of choice in massive PE, however, because of its rapid action. With DVT, subcutaneous unfractionated heparin is an effective alternative. Detailed dosage regimens are given in the RCOG guideline on thromboembolic disease in pregnancy and the puerperium[21], which is also available at www.rcog.org.uk.

Low molecular weigh heparins (LMWH) have been shown in non-pregnant patients to be more effective than unfractionated heparin and warfarin, and to carry a lower risk of haemorrhagic complications[21,24]. They are safe in pregnancy[25,26], have a lower risk of heparin-induced thrombocytopaenia[27] and appear to carry a lower risk of osteoporosis than unfractionated heparin[28,29]. The RCOG guideline recommends a twice-daily dosage regimen, with the exact dose being related to the patient's body weight[21], but a recent systematic review concluded that once daily treatment is as effective as twice-daily treatment[30]. The peak anti-Xa activity should be checked 3 h after injection but frequent monitoring does not appear to be necessary and need not be done until the next routine working day after starting treatment. The platelet count should be checked 7–9 days after starting treatment.

With DVT, the affected leg should be elevated and a graduated compression stocking applied. If the viability of the leg is threatened by DVT or if there is massive life-threatening PE, embolectomy or thrombolytic therapy may be needed. Recurrent PE may indicate insertion of a filter in the inferior vena cava.

Maintenance treatment of DVT or PE

Oral anticoagulants are generally avoided in pregnancy because they cross the placenta. They can cause embryopathy in the first trimester and central nervous system abnormalities at any time during pregnancy, and their anticoagulant effect on the fetus may cause haemorrhagic problems.

Subcutaneous heparin, in the form of either unfractionated heparin or LMWH, can be given for the remainder of the pregnancy, in an adjusted-dose regimen. LMWH are preferable because they are simpler to administer and women can be taught to self-inject. Treatment can be monitored on an outpatient basis, and the platelet count should be checked monthly to detect heparin-induced thrombocytopaenia. Treatment should be continued for at least 6 months and for at least 6–12 weeks after delivery.

Warfarin may be used after delivery. Women taking warfarin may breastfeed without risk to the baby, and the same is probably true for LMWH. Graduated elastic compression stockings should be worn on the affected leg for 2 years after the event, as this substantially reduces the risk of post-thrombotic syndrome. Some authorities have suggested that they should be worn for 5 years after the acute event[31].

Anticoagulant therapy during labour and delivery

During labour, heparin should be given in a thromboprophylactic dose, returning to a therapeutic dose after delivery. Epidural anaesthesia should not be used until at least 12 h after the last prophylactic dose of LMWH[32], or 24 h after the last therapeutic dose. Afterwards, the epidural cannula should not be removed until 10–12 h after the last injection and at least 4 h should then elapse before the next LMWH injection.

For elective caesarean section, the heparin injection should be omitted on the morning of the operation. A prophylactic dose can be given 3–4 h after the operation and a therapeutic dose in the evening. Wound drains should be considered at operation, and the skin closed with interrupted sutures or staples.

Women at high risk of haemorrhage should be treated with intravenous unfractionated heparin, which has a shorter half-life than LMWH and can be more completely reversed with protamine sulphate.

Prevention

The first advance in preventing deaths from VTE was in the 1960s when the importance of early mobilization after normal delivery was recognized. In the 1950s most deaths from VTE occurred after vaginal delivery and the numbers fell when the practice of 'lying in'—enforced bed rest after normal delivery—was abolished.

The next advance was the reduction in deaths from VTE after caesarean section in the UK in the late 1990s[6]. This followed the publication in 1995 of RCOG guidelines on thromboprophylaxis for operative procedures including caesarean section[33]. The number of deaths from postoperative embolism fell from 15 in 1994–6 to four in 1997–9 (Table 2), despite a rise in the caesarean section rate[34]. Table 3 shows that there was no increase in the number of late deaths, indicating that VTE deaths after caesarean section were not merely being delayed.

This dramatic improvement suggested that deaths from thromboembolism can be prevented if women at risk are identified and guidelines on prophylaxis are followed. Guidelines for thromboprophylaxis in vaginal deliveries were included in *Why Mothers Die 1997–1999*[6], and in June 2003, the RCOG published draft guidelines for thromboprophylaxis during pregnancy and after normal delivery[35].

The key to prevention, as with diagnosis, is awareness of the condition. Recent reports of the UK Confidential Enquiries into Maternal Deaths have raised awareness of thromboembolism and especially of risk factors. Of the 31 women whose deaths were reported in 1997–1999, obvious risk factors were present in 25 cases[36]. Thirteen women were overweight, five had had a period of bed rest, four had a family history, three had previous thromboembolism, two had undertaken long-haul flights during pregnancy and one had varicose veins. Some had multiple risk factors. In addition, 18 of the women were aged over 30.

Of the six women with no recorded risk factors, five died before 25 weeks' gestation. Thrombophilia may have been a factor in these deaths. Five of the late deaths were associated with the oral contraceptive pill: all five women were overweight and in two their obesity should have contraindicated the combined pill[36].

Risk assessment and thromboprophylaxis

All women should undergo an assessment of their risk for VTE, ideally before pregnancy, or failing that, in early pregnancy. Risk is high in the first trimester and death may occur before the antenatal booking visit. The assessment should be repeated if the woman is admitted to hospital or develops other problems.

LMWH is effective for thromboprophylaxis in pregnancy[37]. The draft RCOG guideline suggests that a woman with three or more of the risk factors in Table 4 should receive prophylactic LMWH antenatally and for at least 3–5 days postpartum. A woman with two or more risk factors should receive prophylactic LMWH for 3–5 days after normal delivery.

Careful enquiry should be made about a past history or a family history of VTE. A woman with a previous VTE should undergo screening for thrombophilia, ideally before pregnancy. If thrombophilia is excluded, the question of antenatal thromboprophylaxis is controversial. It is generally felt that if the previous VTE was provoked by a temporary risk factor (such as immobilization or trauma) which has now resolved, thromboprophylaxis is not necessary antenatally, though it should be given postpartum.

A woman with a previous VTE and a family history in a first-degree relative should receive antenatal thromboprophylaxis with LMWH. The same applies to a woman with recurrent VTE. A family history suggests thrombophilia. Women with a previous VTE who have thrombophilia should receive antenatal and postpartum thromboprophylaxis.

Antenatal screening of all women for thrombophilia has been suggested but has not proven effective[38]. A large number of women will screen 'positive' and it is unrealistic to recommend thromboprophylaxis to a high proportion of healthy pregnant women. Nevertheless, women may present in pregnancy with no personal history of VTE but with a known thrombophilia. Again, the risk of VTE depends on the specific thrombophilia. Antithrombin deficiency carries a 30% risk of VTE in pregnancy. Protein C or protein S deficiency carries an eight-fold increase in risk—mainly of postpartum VTE. Heterozygotes for factor V Leiden are at

Table 4 Risk factors for venous thromboembolism in pregnancy and the puerperium

Pre-existing	New onset/transient
Previous VTE	Surgical procedure in pregnancy or puerperium
Family history of VTE	Immobility (>4 days bed rest)
Obesity (BMI >30 kg/m²)	Hyperemesis
Thrombophilia	Dehydration
Congenital	Ovarian hyperstimulation syndrome
Antithrombin deficiency	Infection (*e.g.* UTI)
Protein C deficiency	Pre-eclampsia
Protein S deficiency	Excessive blood loss
Factor V Leiden	Long haul air travel
Prothrombin gene variant	Prolonged labour
Acquired (antiphospholipid syndrome)	
Lupus anticoagulant	
Anticardiolipin antibodies	
Age over 35 years	
Parity greater than 4	
Gross varicose veins	
Paraplegia	
Sickle cell disease	
Inflammatory disorders, *e.g.* inflammatory bowel disease	
Some medical conditions, *e.g.* nephrotic syndrome, some cardiac diseases	

Adapted from draft RCOG guideline[35].

considerably lower risk. Antenatal thromboprophylaxis is not usually necessary except in those with combined defects, those homozygous for defects, or those with antithrombin deficiency. All women with thrombophilia should, however, receive LMWH or warfarin for 6 weeks after delivery.

In antiphospholipid syndrome (lupus anticoagulant or anticardiolipin antibodies associated with thrombosis or adverse pregnancy outcome), the risk of recurrent thromboses may be 70% or even higher. Pregnant women with antiphospholipid syndrome and previous thrombosis should receive antenatal and postnatal thromboprophylaxis with LMWH. This is not required for women with anticardiolipin antibodies and no history of thrombosis or pregnancy loss.

Timing and duration of thromboprophylaxis

Thromboprophylaxis should begin as early as practicable in pregnancy and should continue until delivery. LMWH should be continued during labour and delivery because of the high risk of initiation of VTE immediately after delivery. For epidural or caesarean section, however, and for women at high risk of haemorrhage, the guidance given in the section on treatment should be followed.

Postpartum thromboprophylaxis should be started as soon as possible after delivery, provided there is no postpartum haemorrhage. LMWH should be started 3 h after delivery (or 4 h after removal of an epidural catheter). Thromboprophylaxis is normally continued for 6 weeks in high risk women, as it takes several weeks for the prothrombotic changes of pregnancy to revert to normal. For women at lower risk (*e.g.* those with obesity or age >35), prophylaxis for 3–5 days after delivery is usually recommended.

Puerperal women undergoing surgery or travelling by air are at increased risk of VTE. The RCOG has issued advice for pregnant women travelling by air: for those already at increased risk and undertaking long-haul flights LMWH is recommended but low-dose aspirin is an acceptable alternative if LMWH is impractical to administer[36,39].

Agents for prophylaxis

LMWH are preferred to unfractionated heparin for thromboprophylaxis. Dosages are given in the RCOG guideline (available at www.rcog.org.uk). If renal function is normal, monitoring of anti-Xa levels is not necessary, except in antithrombin deficiency. Low dose aspirin may be appropriate when the risk of VTE is not high enough to warrant antenatal LMWH, for example in women without thrombophilia but with previous VTE due to a specific cause. Warfarin is suitable for prolonged postpartum thromboprophylaxis. Dextran carries a risk of anaphylaxis and should not be used. Danaparoid has been used in case of heparin-induced thrombocytopaenia[40].

All women with previous VTE or thrombophilia should be encouraged to wear graduated elastic compression stockings throughout pregnancy and for 6–12 weeks after delivery, though strong evidence for this recommendation is lacking. The use of such stockings is also recommended for pregnant women travelling by air.

Conclusion

For many years, maternal death from thromboembolism was thought to be sudden and unavoidable. Better understanding of the clinical presentation and risk factors, along with the development of more convenient methods of diagnosis and treatment, and in particular the publication of detailed guidelines for thromboprophylaxis for women at risk, open up the possibility of making a real reduction in this cause of maternal mortality and morbidity.

References

1 Tovey C, Wyatt S. Diagnosis, investigation, and management of deep vein thrombosis. *BMJ* 2003; **326**: 1180–4

2 Rosendaal FR. Venous thrombosis: a multicausal disease. *Lancet* 1999; **353**: 1167–73

3 British National Formulary 39. London: British Medical Association and Royal Pharmaceutical Society of Great Britian, 2001

4 Simpson EL, Lawrenson RA, Nightingale AL, Farmer RD. Venous thromboembolism in pregnancy and the puerperium: incidence and additional risk factors from a London perinatal database. *Br J Obstet Gynaecol* 2001; **108**: 56–60

5 Greer IA. Thrombosis in pregnancy: maternal and fetal issues. *Lancet* 1999; **353**: 1258–65

6 Lewis G (ed) *Why Mothers Die 1997–1999. Report of the Confidential Enquiry into Maternal Deaths in the UK*. London: RCOG Press, 2001

7 Drife JO. The third generation pill controversy ('continued'). *BMJ* 2001; **323**: 119–20

8 Drife J. Oral contraception and the risk of thromboembolism. What does it mean to clinicians and their patients? *Drug Safety* 2002; **25**: 893–902

9 Geelhoed DW, Visser LE, Asare K, Schagen van Leeuwen JH, van Roosmalen J. Trends in maternal mortality: a 13-year study in rural Ghana. *Eur J Obstet Gynecol Reprod Biol* 2003; **107**: 135–9

10 Pattinson R (ed) *Saving Mothers 1999–2001. Second Report on Confidential Enquiries into Maternal Deaths in South Africa*. www.doh.gov.za

11 Kilpatrick SJ, Crabtree KE, Kemp A, Geller S. Preventability of maternal deaths: comparison between Zambian and American referral hospitals. *Obstet Gynecol* 2002; **100**: 321–6

12 Berg CJ, Chang J, Callaghan WM, Whitehead SJ. Pregnancy-related mortality in the United States, 1991–1997. *Obstet Gynecol* 2003; **101**: 289–96

13 Salanave B, Bouvier-Colle M-H, Varnoux N, Alexander S, Macfarlane A and the MOMS Group. Classification differences and maternal mortality: a European study. *Int J Epidemiol* 1999; **28**: 64–9

14 Schuitemaker N, Van Roosmalen J, Dekker G, Van Dongen P, Van Geijn H, Gravenhorst JB. Underreporting of maternal mortality in the Netherlands. *Obstet Gynecol* 1997; **90**: 78–82

15 Department of Health and Social Security. *Report on Confidential Enquiries into Maternal Deaths in England and Wales 1976–1978*. London: Her Majesty's Stationery Office, 1982

16 Department of Health. *Report on Confidential Enquiries into Maternal Deaths in England and Wales 1982–84*. London: Her Majesty's Stationery Office, 1989

17 Jilma B, Kamath S, Lip GYH. Antithrombotic therapy in special circumstances. II. In children, thrombophilia, and miscellaneous conditions. *BMJ* 2003; **326**: 93–6

18 Killewich LA, Martin R, Cramer M, Beach KW, Strandness DE. An objective assessment of the physiological changes in the postthrombotic syndrome. *Arch Surg* 1985; **120**: 424–6

19 Kahn SR, Hirsch A, Shrier I. Effect of postthrombotic syndrome on health-related quality of life after deep venous thrombosis. *Arch Intern Med* 2002; **162**: 1144–8

20 Chan WS, Ginsberg JS. Diagnosis of deep vein thrombosis and pulmonary embolism in pregnancy. *Thromb Res* 2002; **107**: 85–91

21 Royal College of Obstetricians and Gynaecologists. *Thromboembolic Disease in Pregnancy and the Puerperium: Acute Management*. Clinical Green Top Guideline No. 28. London: RCOG Press, 2001

22 Janata K. Managing pulmonary embolism. *BMJ* 2003; **326**: 1341–2

23 Turpie AGG, Chin BSP, Lip GYH. Venous thromboembolism: treatment strategies. *BMJ* 2002; **325**: 948–50

24 Working Group on behalf of the Obstetric Medicine Group of Australasia. Anticoagulation in pregnancy and the puerperium. *Med J Aust* 2001; **175**: 258–63

25 Eldor A. The use of low-molecular-weight heparin for the management of venous thromboembolism in pregnancy. *Eur J Obstet Gynecol Reprod Biol* 2002; **104**: 3–13

26 Lepercq J, Conard J, Borel-Derlon A *et al*. Venous thromboembolism during pregnancy: a retrospective study of enoxaparin safety in 624 pregnancies. *Br J Obstet Gynaecol* 2001; **108**: 1134–40

27 Blann AD, Landray MJ, Lip GYH. An overview of antithrombotic therapy. *BMJ* 2002; **325**: 762–5

28   Jilma B, Kamath S, Lip GYH. Antithrombotic therapy in special circumstances. I—pregnancy and cancer. *BMJ* 2003; **326**: 37–40

29   Rodie VA, Thomson AJ, Stewart FM, Quinn AJ, Walker LD, Greer IA. Low molecular weight heparin for the treatment of venous thromboembolism in pregnancy: a case series. *Br J Obstet Gynaecol* 2002; **109**: 1020–4

30   van Dongen CJ, MacGillavry MR, Prins MH. Once versus twice daily LMWH for the initial treatment of venous thromboembolism (Cochrane Review). In: *The Cochrane Library, Issue 2, 2003.* Oxford: Update Software

31   Franzeck UK, Schalch I, Bollinger A. On the relationship between changes in the deep veins evaluated by duplex sonography and the postthrombotic syndrome 12 years after deep vein thrombosis. *Thromb Haemost* 1997; **77**: 1109–12

32   Crossley D, Zych Z. Timing of thromboprophylaxis for general surgery should be discussed with anaesthetists. *BMJ* 2000; **321**: 1018

33   Royal College of Obstetricians and Gynaecologists. *Report of a Working Party on Prophylaxis against Thromboembolism in Gynaecology and Obstetrics.* London: RCOG Press, 1995

34   The National Sentinel Caesarean Section Audit Report. London: RCOG Clinical Effectiveness Support Unit, 2001

35   Royal College of Obstetricians and Gynaecologists. *Guideline: Thromboprophylaxis During Pregnancy and After Normal Vaginal Delivery.* London: RCOG Press, 2003

36   Drife J on behalf of the Editorial Board. Thrombosis and thromboembolism. In: Lewis G (ed) *Why Mothers Die 1997–1999. Report of the Confidential Enquiry into Maternal Deaths in the UK.* London: RCOG Press, 2001; 49–75

37   Hunt BJ, Doughty HA, Majumdar G, Copplestone A, Kerslake S, Buchanan N, Hughes G, Khamashta M. Thromboprophylaxis with low molecular weight heparin (Fragmin) in high risk pregnancies. *Thromb Haemost* 1997; **77**: 39–43

38   Lindqvist PG, Olofsson P, Dahlback B. Use of selective Factor V Leiden screening in pregnancy to identify candidates for anticoagulants. *Obstet Gynecol* 2002; **100**: 332–6

39   Royal College of Obstetricians and Gynaecologists. *Advice on Preventing Deep Vein Thrombosis for Pregnant Women Travelling by Air.* Scientific Advisory Committee Opinion Paper 1. London: RCOG Press, 2001

40   Woo YL, Allard S, Cohen H, Letsky E, de Swiet M. Danaparoid thromboprophylaxis in pregnant women with heparin-induced thrombocytopenia. *Br J Obstet Gynaecol* 2002; **109**: 466–8

Obstructed labour

JP Neilson*, **T Lavender†**, **S Quenby*** and **S Wray‡**

*Departments of *Obstetrics & Gynaecology and ‡Physiology, University of Liverpool, Liverpool and †Department of Midwifery Studies, University of Central Lancashire, Preston, UK*

Obstructed labour is an important cause of maternal deaths in communities in which undernutrition in childhood is common resulting in small pelves in women, and in which there is no easy access to functioning health facilities with the capability of carrying out operative deliveries. Obstructed labour also causes significant maternal morbidity in the short term (notably infection) and long term (notably obstetric fistulas). Fetal death from asphyxia is also common. There are differences in the behaviour of the uterus during obstructed labour, depending on whether the woman has delivered previously. The pattern in primigravid women (typically diminishing contractility with risk of infection and fistula) may result from tissue acidosis, whereas in parous women, contractility may be maintained with the risk of uterine rupture. Ultimately, tackling the problem of obstructed labour will require universal adequate nutritional intake from childhood and the ability to access adequately equipped and staffed clinical facilities when problems arise in labour. These seem still rather distant aspirations. In the meantime, strategies should be implemented to encourage early recognition of prolonged labour and appropriate clinical responses. The sequelae of obstructed labour can be an enormous source of human misery and the prevention of obstetric fistulas, and skilled treatment if they do occur, are important priorities in regions where obstructed labour is still common.

Introduction

Correspondence to:
Prof. JP Neilson,
University Department of
Obstetrics & Gynaecology,
Liverpool Women's
Hospital, Crown Street,
Liverpool L8 7SS, UK.
E-mail: jneilson@liv.ac.uk

Each year, 210 million women become pregnant, of whom 20 million will experience pregnancy-related illness and 500,000 will die as a result of the complications of pregnancy or childbirth[1]. In 1987, the World Health Organization (WHO) launched the Safe Motherhood Initiative, which aimed to reduce maternal morbidity and mortality by 50% by the year 2000. The initiative did not succeed but maternal health continues to be a major focus of WHO effort. The current WHO initiative[2] is to reduce maternal mortality to 75% of the 1990 level by 2015. If this is to be successful, the problem of obstructed labour will need to be addressed effectively.

British Medical Bulletin 2003; **67**: 191–204
DOI: 10.1093/bmb/ldg018

Obstructed labour remains an important cause of not only maternal death but also short- and long-term disability. It has particular impact in communities in which mechanical problems during labour are common and availability of functioning relevant health services is sparse. Obstructed labour comprises one of the five major causes of maternal mortality and morbidity in developing countries[3,4]. The number of maternal deaths as a result of obstructed labour and/or rupture of the uterus varies between 4% and 70% of all maternal deaths, amounting to a maternal mortality rate as high as 410/100,000 live births[5]. The literature suggests that in many countries, maternal mortality due to this cause is almost as prevalent today as it was 30 years ago.

Maternal mortality from obstructed labour is largely the result of ruptured uterus or puerperal infection, whereas perinatal mortality is mainly due to asphyxia. Significant maternal morbidity is associated with prolonged labour, since both post-partum haemorrhage and infection are more common in women with long labours. Obstetric fistulas are long-term problems. Traumatic delivery affects both mother and child.

In this paper, we will describe important epidemiological associations of obstructed labour, its definition, recognition and management, and chart the serious sequelae that may follow—especially if clinical intervention is tardy or inappropriate or, as is commonly the case in much of the world, simply unavailable. We will also speculate on why there are differences in the behaviour of the uterus in women who have obstructed labour and who have, or have not, had babies previously—based on emerging but incomplete understandings of the cellular physiology and pathophysiology of uterine contractility.

Definitions

The term 'obstructed labour' indicates a failure to progress due to mechanical problems—a mismatch between fetal size, or more accurately, the size of the presenting part of the fetus, and the mother's pelvis, although some malpresentations, notably a brow presentation or a shoulder presentation (the latter in association with a transverse lie) will also cause obstruction. Pathological enlargement of the fetal head, as in hydrocephalus, may also (though rarely) obstruct labour. Difficult labour may also be associated with an occipito-posterior position of the fetal head and with ineffective uterine contractions (the latter often described as 'dysfunctional labour'). These different causes of dystocia (difficult labour) may co-exist.

Epidemiology

There is a substantial literature, reviewed elsewhere[6], to show an association between cephalo-pelvic disproportion, as a cause of obstructed labour, and maternal height—which is linked to pelvic size. Maternal height reflects the nutritional status of individuals from childhood. There may be large deviations from normal if there had been rickets in childhood or osteomalacia in adolescence. Pregnancy in adolescence may pose problems even without gross nutritional deficiencies because the bony pelvis may not yet have achieved its full dimensions. Different cut-off heights have been identified in different communities to highlight an increased risk of obstetric labour, the individual values reflecting genetic diversity[6].

Consequences

The risk of maternal death from obstructed labour is greatest in developing countries with poorly resourced health services. Most reports come from tertiary referral, specialist hospitals and the findings of case series in these institutions may not reflect the reality in the community. However, a community-based retrospective survey of maternal deaths in a region of Uganda, using the sisterhood method, found 26% of 324 deaths to be attributable to obstructed labour[7]; this cause was second only to haemorrhage. A similar proportion (19% of 350 deaths) was identified in a prospective study, using verbal autopsies, in Guinea-Bissau[8].

In communities with poor access to obstetric care, obstructed labour leads to maternal dehydration, infection, ketosis and exhaustion. The major immediate causes of death in obstructed labour are sepsis, and haemorrhage from uterine rupture. Sepsis is more common in primigravid women, and uterine rupture in parous women. It is commonly observed that obstruction in the primigravid woman is associated with a gradual decrease in the strength and frequency of contractions, whilst obstruction in the parous woman does not seem to decrease contractility so that the lower segment continues to thin until rupture occurs. We speculate on the possible reasons for this later. Sepsis results from the prolonged state of an open cervix often with ruptured membranes impairing natural, mechanical barriers to ascending infection from the vagina.

Obstructed labour is the leading cause of uterine rupture worldwide. It is very rare in primigravid labours. A recent 7 year review carried out in Ghana found that rupture was due to prolonged labour in around one-third of all cases[9]. Similar figures have been reported from other regions (e.g. in Delhi 27% of ruptures in a 5 year period were due to obstructed labour[10]). Uterine rupture is life threatening because of the haemorrhage, and is often treated by total abdominal hysterectomy. The perinatal mortality rate in the above studies was around 75% and maternal deaths in these teaching hospitals were 1 and 3%. Higher values will occur in less well resourced areas; a study, for example, examining obstetrical causes of maternal morbidity in six West African countries, reported obstructed labour as being, like the Uganda study, second only to haemorrhage as a cause of maternal morbidity with a fatality rate of 30% attributed to poor obstetrical care[11].

Women who have undergone caesarean section previously for obstructed labour are particularly at risk of uterine rupture in subsequent labours, especially if stimulated by uterotonic drugs, or if remote from clinical facilities.

Fistula formation is more common in the primigravid woman. In a large case series from the famous fistula hospital in Addis Abada, 97% of vesico-vaginal fistulas occurred after obstructed labour; 65% of women were aged less than 25; and 63% had been primigravid[12]. Vesico-vaginal fistulas mainly result from the ischaemic necrosis of vaginal and bladder tissues, trapped between the fetal head and the mother's pubic symphysis during prolonged, obstructed labour. Recto-vaginal fistulas may also form but these are less common, presumably because of the absence of a maternal bony surface in close proximity, posteriorly. Uncontrollable passage of urine, and sometimes faeces, through the vagina assures a wretched existence[13]. There is, in addition, damage to a wider field of pelvic tissue than that which necroses and sloughs to form the fistula, resulting potentially in urethral and cervical destruction, stress incontinence, vaginal stenosis, amenorrhoea, osteitis pubis and foot-drop[14].

Physiology of uterine contractions

Consideration of the different types of adverse outcome in primigravid and parous women in obstructed labour requires review of what is known about the physiology of uterine contractility.

Once initiated, labour consists of a series of uterine contractions. Typically these will last for 60 s and reach pressures of 50 mmHg. This represents a significant metabolic demand upon the mother. Our knowledge of the mechanisms underlying the contractions has increased considerably in the last decade. There is a pattern of electrical changes, depolarization, across the membrane of the smooth muscle cells in the uterus, which opens channels permeable to calcium. On entering the myometrial cell, the calcium binds to calmodulin and activates the enzyme myosin light chain kinase (MLCK). Activated MLCK phosphorylates myosin, thereby stimulating interaction with actin and subsequent cross-bridge cycling and contraction. The cross-bridge cycle consumes ATP and ATP hydrolysis produces acidification. This basic cycle of:

$$depolarization \longrightarrow \uparrow Ca^{2+} \longrightarrow active\ MLCK \longrightarrow contraction$$

can be modified by agents occurring naturally or administered clinically, such as oxytocin and prostaglandins. For example oxytocin can augment the rise in calcium, decrease the rate of calcium efflux from the cell and decrease the rate at which myosin is dephosphorylated (and inactivated). All these effects will promote stronger and longer contractions.

Physiologically, the uterus has been prepared for labour by altering the expression and control of those proteins needed for contraction. In particular, the balance of the ion channels shifts, so that potassium channels, which are associated with hyperpolarization, are less influential on the membrane potential. This in turn will increase the chance of the calcium channels opening and increase the contractile drive on the uterus. Biochemically, the myometrium has also been preparing for labour by increasing its glycogen store and fatty acid droplets. There is also a small increase in phosphocreatine, from which ATP can be re-formed from ADP. Lactate dehydrogenase also increases its activity, so that more pyruvate will be formed into lactic acid, rather than entering the Kreb's cycle for oxidative metabolism. These changes can be summarized as a preparation for periods of anaerobic metabolism. This is exactly what happens in labour, as the powerful contractions compress uterine blood vessels, causing transient hypoxic episodes. The myometrium responds by producing ATP anaerobically, *i.e. via* lactic acid, and utilizing its reserves.

There appear to be fundamental differences between the behaviour of the uterus of the primigravid women and the parous women in obstructed labour. Rupture, rather than fistula, appears as a more common consequence in parous women. We can find no clear descriptions of uterine activity during obstructed labours. It appears that in primigravid women, if a mechanical obstruction to labour exists, the uterine contractions gradually weaken and then stop. However, in multiparous women, contractions continue until delivery or uterine rupture occurs.

Pathophysiology of uterine contractions in obstructed labour

The obvious purpose of labour is to deliver the fetus and then placenta, whether the labour becomes obstructed or not. Thus, the initial pattern of uterine activity will be the same in the two cases. The uterus will expend energy producing cycles of contraction and relaxation. The metabolic cost of this can be met in a healthy mother and activity sustained for many hours. However, if the hours become days then the situation will change. Leaving aside for the moment the emotional distress and physical exhaustion of the mother, along with the restricted intake of food and drink, what will be happening to the uterus? It will gradually be depleting its metabolic reserves, *i.e.* glycogen, and finding difficulty in maintaining ATP levels. There may also be an acidification due to the continued production of lactic acid coupled with a decreased ability to extrude protons, as this is energetically demanding and ultimately relies on ATP. We know from work on animal and human uteri that acidification decreases the ability of the uterus to contract. Therefore it is not difficult to predict that uterine contractions will start to weaken in prolonged labours, due to physiological and biochemical reasons.

Therefore, we can propose a hypothesis for diminished uterine contractility in obstructed labour in primigravid women. The uterus probably stops contracting because of myometrial acidification. This acidification results from local myometrial energy depletion, anaerobic metabolism, and systemic ketosis. In parous women, perhaps the myometrium becomes tolerant to the effects of acidification by an unknown mechanism and does not stop contracting. Continued contractions in the presence of myometrial energy depletion and hypoxia are likely to lead to myometrial oedema and necrosis contributing to uterine rupture.

In addition to optimizing the clinical care of women with obstructed labour, there is an urgent need for high quality research to link clinical observations and intervention studies to the laboratory sciences. The questions remaining to be addressed if the WHO objectives are to be achieved are: an accurate definition of obstructed labour, verification of the pathophysiology of obstructed labour and the prevention of consequences arising from obstructed labour.

Recognition and prevention of prolonged labour

Improved outcome after obstructed labour requires early detection of abnormal progress of labour, and appropriate clinical responses in accessible, equipped and staffed units. Before the problems of preventing and managing prolonged labour can be addressed, it is first important to highlight the difficulties of defining exactly what constitutes an abnormal labour.

Confirmation of progress in labour is determined by the identification of increasing cervical dilatation and cervical effacement. Normal labour has been defined as when a baby is born within a period of 12 h, *via* the natural passages, through the efforts of the mother, and when no harm befalls either party as a result of the experience[15]. Yet, a more useful definition is the rate of progress of cervical dilatation (usually expressed in centimetres per hour)[16]. Correction of prolonged labour is therefore dependent on regular cervical assessment. However, this measure, although generally accepted, may not be precise and there are no reported trials of either inter-observer or intra-observer reproducibility.

Midwives and obstetricians can all agree that a major degree of cephalo-pelvic disproportion should be classified as abnormal[17]. However, there is little consensus concerning the labouring primigravida who has made slow but steady progress for, say, 20 h in the absence of maternal or fetal distress. The definition of normality is vague, with a resulting variation in hospital guidelines. Many studies have described the duration and velocity of labour in various groups of women ranging from a normal duration of labour for a primigravida being 5.6 h[18] to suggestions that 13.3 h is more appropriate[19]. Yet these data lack clinical relevance, as direct comparisons are difficult owing to variations in study eligibility criteria. A more recent definition of prolonged labour provided by WHO for primiparous women was more than 18 h[5]. In contrast, in the National Maternity Hospital in Dublin, the definition of a prolonged labour has been steadily and systematically reduced from 48 to 12 h[20]. In the struggle to balance early diagnosis and correction of prolonged labour with the use of unnecessary intervention, no consensus has yet been reached amongst midwives and obstetricians to provide a definition of normality.

History of the partogram

The development of the partograph (or partogram) provided health professionals with a pictorial overview of the labour to allow early identification and diagnosis of the pathological labour.

The first obstetrician to provide a realistic tool for the study of individual labours was Emanuel Friedman[21]. In his study of 100 primigravidae at term, cervical dilatation was determined by frequent rectal examinations. For reproducibility, the examination was carried out at the peak of the contraction and for uniformity, measurements were recorded in centimetres. A simple, but effective chart was devised whereby square graph paper was used, with 10 divisions representing the cervical dilatation. The measurements were recorded and joined to the previous measurement in a straight line. The slope of each line was determined in terms of centimetres of dilatation per hour. The curves obtained by this simple technique were similar in shape and resembled a sigmoid curve. Friedman's explanation divided the first stage of labour into two parts: firstly, the latent phase which extends over 8–10 h and up to 3 cm dilatation; secondly, the active phase, characterized by acceleration from 3 to 10 cm, at the end of which is a decelerative phase. The major criticism of the development of this curve was the fact that no exclusions were made for malpresentations, malpositions or multiple pregnancies. Similarly, women receiving oxytocin infusions, caudal analgesia and/or operative delivery were included. However, although the Friedman's labour curve is a crude version of the one used by many midwives and obstetricians today, it did recognize the fact that labour is sensitive to interference, prolonged with heavy sedation and shortened with stimulation. These have remained important factors when managing labouring women.

A randomized study of 434 women in Mexico[22] reinforces the benefits of the Friedman partogram. In this study, women were randomized to either a Friedman partogram or a non-graphical descriptive chart. The results showed that there were more operative deliveries in the descriptive group and more babies with low Apgar scores at 5 min. The conclusions drawn from this study were that the Friedman partogram not only has diagnostic and prognostic value but that it also benefits the management of women in labour.

Philpott's partograph developed from the original cervicograph of Friedman, providing a practical tool for recording intrapartum details[23]. This was in an attempt to rationalize the use of maternity services in Harare (then Salisbury) in Zimbabwe (then Rhodesia). This structure has been replicated elsewhere in the developing world and comprised a hospital with medical staff and operating theatre facilities, and 13 peripheral clinics staffed mainly by midwives. Approximately half of the 40,000 deliveries took place in the hospital and it was imperative to ensure that only high risk women delivered there.

To advance Friedman's partograph, an alert line was placed on the cervicograph. This innovation was introduced following the results of a prospective study of 624 consecutive women[24]. Unlike Friedman, Philpott and Castle had a more focused eligibility criteria for their study. Women were only included in the study if the cervix was already 3 cm dilated on admission.

The alert line, unlike that of Friedman's, was straight, not curved. The line was a modification of the mean rate of cervical dilatation of the slowest 10% of primigravid women in the active phase of labour and progressed at a rate of 1 cm per hour. Should a woman's cervical dilatation progress slowly and cross the 'transfer line', 2 h to the right of the alert line, then arrangements were made to transfer her from a peripheral unit to the central unit where prolonged labour could be managed more effectively.

The next stage in the development of the partogram by Philpott and Castle was the introduction of an action line drawn 4 h to the right of the alert line[24]. This line was developed on the premise that correction of primary inefficient uterine action would lead to a vaginal delivery. To evaluate the action line, a prospective study was carried out which concluded that the action line allowed 50% of patients whose cervicograph crossed the alert line to avoid being given oxytocin stimulation. It also showed a lowered incidence of prolonged labour and a reduction in caesarean sections. However, the reliability of this study can be questioned as although it is a 'prospective clinical study of 624 patients', many of the findings are based on a comparison of women who delivered in the department in 1966. Furthermore, the actual number of women who crossed the action line was only 68; chance findings can therefore not be completely excluded.

What is surprising perhaps is that the use of the partogram itself was only rigorously evaluated 20 years after its introduction[5]. The WHO partogram is an adaptation of the one formulated and described by Philpott and colleagues. To test whether the use of the WHO partograph improves labour management and reduces maternal and fetal morbidity and mortality, a prospective study of 35,484 women was carried out. The study lasted 15 months and involved four pairs of tertiary level hospitals in South East Asia. During the first 5 months all the hospitals collected data about delivery. For the next 5 months the WHO partograph was introduced into one of each hospital pair. For the last 5 months, the partograph was introduced into the remaining four hospitals. The protocol for management of labour included no intervention in the latent phase until after 8 h, amniotomy in the active phase, augmentation, caesarean section or observation to be considered if the action line is reached. The introduction of this package was accompanied by 'several days' of intensive teaching of the midwifery and the medical staff. The outcomes that showed significant improvement were: fewer prolonged labours (>18 h), fewer augmented labours and less post-partum sepsis.

In order to avoid the pitfalls of a historical control design, hospitals were randomly allocated to implement the partograph in phases. However, this method also had its pitfalls. The authors state that it was not possible to randomize the individual to either conventional or to partograph care. There is only one reliable way of testing whether an intervention improves outcome and that is with a randomized controlled trial. The research method used in that study had several ways in which the results could have been biased and lays the results open to doubt.

To test whether the partograph was the cause of change in outcome between the hospitals studied, the introduction of the partogram should have been the only variable which was changed. In this study, the introduction of the partogram was accompanied by several days intensive teaching of midwifery and medical staff with the help of a WHO consultant in each centre. It was also introduced with a protocol, which specified, among other things, that the women's membranes were ruptured in the active phase of labour. Either, or both of these latter changes could have led to the change in outcomes, *e.g.* fewer augmented labours.

Even if the results could be relied upon, one could question how applicable they are in other settings, *i.e.* other than in tertiary level hospitals in South East Asia. The authors stated that the WHO trial has shown beyond doubt that the partograph should be used on all women in labour[5]. Yet the effect of the partograph in, for example, a health centre with no facilities for caesarean section and inadequate supplies or a hospital where highly trained midwives give care is uncertain. Thus, the results of this study do not offer adequate support to allow the partograph to be recommended for use for all women.

The WHO press release claims that the use of the partograph reduces the caesarean section rate—in fact, the paper shows that this was not a significant result. Only reductions in prolonged labour, augmented labours and post-partum sepsis reached statistical significance. The authors report that the proportion of labours requiring oxytocic augmentation was reduced by 54%—from 20.7 to 9.1%. It is difficult to come to any conclusion except that the previous rate of augmentation was unnecessarily high. This interpretation is supported by the authors' observation that the improvements were 'most marked in normal women'. In which case, the partograph is simply correcting a poor standard of care, rather than making childbirth safer *per se*.

It must be understood that the majority of trials of partography have taken place in hospital settings where most maternal deaths occur among women admitted with severe complications and often neglected labour[25]. No trial to date (even the WHO trial) has demonstrated that the partograph does reduce maternal mortality.

The partogram as a whole needs to be evaluated further, as do its individual components. There is a need to clarify the association of abnormal patterns with underlying causes. The classical pattern attributed to cephalo-pelvic disproportion is secondary arrest of cervical dilatation, with a normal initial dilatation rate of cervical dilatation followed by cessation of dilatation. However, the situation can undoubtedly be more complex with, for example, relative disproportion being exacerbated by occipito-posterior positions, or secondary failure of uterine contractility occurring with prolonged labour (as described previously). The importance of the observation of degrees of moulding of the fetal head also merits further study.

Management of prolonged labour

It is ironic that in many parts of the western world, there are concerns about caesarean section rates steadily rising without evidence of a reduction in perinatal mortality and morbidity. In contrast, in many parts of the developing world, women with a clear need for operative delivery are not able to access this.

O'Driscoll and Meagher seemed to have discovered the perfect solution to prolonged labour by introducing an 'active management' package[15], which maintained a low caesarean section rate envied by many. Caesarean section rates of 5–7% led to worldwide interest in what has been known as the Dublin Approach. This active management package has become synonymous with early use of amniotomy and syntocinon to achieve a rate of cervical dilatation of at least 1 cm/h. The protocol also depended on accurate diagnosis of labour, a constant support person, the recognition of a latent and active phase in the second stage of labour and peer reviewed audits.

The active management package also places a large emphasis on a high level of support during labour, a factor which has been shown in other studies to be associated with shorter labours, higher rates of normal vaginal delivery and a reduction in the analgesia used[26]. Klaus et al speculated that increased levels of adrenaline are associated with anxiety and prolonged duration of labour[26]. Therefore, social support may lessen anxiety, reducing adrenaline concentrations and thus shortening labour. These Guatemalan studies could be criticized due to the unrepresentative study samples but further, more representative studies have, however, confirmed both the short- and long-term benefits of constant companionship in labour[27].

Clinical trials to test the active management approach are few. Meta-analysis of the randomized clinical trials on specific components of active management shows that oxytocin augmentation does not improve caesarean section rates, operative vaginal delivery rates or neonatal outcome[28], but does increase hyperstimulation and the amount of pain experienced by the woman[29]. Amniotomy, although showing a minimal reduction in labour duration, does not appear to affect perinatal outcome or operative delivery rates[30].

Randomized studies to evaluate the efficacy of the whole package of active management are extremely rare. One study which did appear to assess all aspects of the active management package was that carried out by Frigoletto et al[31]. This study was probably the first to provide enough evidence to forcefully challenge the management as outlined by the Dublin group. Frigoletto randomly assigned 1934 nulliparous low risk women to either an active management group or usual-care group, before 30 weeks gestation. The components of active management were identical to those outlined by O'Driscoll et al in Dublin[20]: customized childbirth classes; strict criteria for labour diagnosis; standardized labour management (which included early amniotomy and treatment with high dose oxytocin); and one-to-one nursing support.

Women with full-term, uncomplicated pregnancies who presented in spontaneous labour (the protocol-eligible subgroup), who had been assigned to the active management group were admitted to a separate unit.

Despite the 'active management package', no differences were found between groups in the rate of caesarean section, either among all women or in the protocol-eligible subgroup. However, the median duration of labour was shorter in the protocol-eligible subgroup by 2.7 h and the rate of maternal fever was lower (7% *versus* 11%, P = 0.007). There were three times as many women whose labour lasted more than 12 h in the usual-care group than in the active management group (26% *versus* 9%, P < 0.001). From this study, one may conclude that active management of labour may not reduce caesarean section rates but it may be associated with some outcomes which may be considered as favourable. Frigoletto *et al* do acknowledge the possibility of the Hawthorne effect contributing to their findings. That is, because they were focused on caesarean section rates, the overall caesarean section rate was reduced. They did evaluate this potential effect retrospectively and found no differences in mode of delivery and oxytocin use between the usual-care group who were protocol-eligible and all low risk women who delivered their first baby during the 6 months preceding trial commencement. The conclusion from Frigoletto *et al* was that their data do not provide adequate justification for the universal recommendation of active management of labour. Their study contributes to the many controversial debates surrounding labour management.

Operative delivery

When there is clear evidence of obstruction in the first stage of labour, delivery by caesarean section is usually required. A number of Cochrane systematic reviews, completed or in progress, assess the best evidence for different techniques. Antibiotic prophylaxis is important[32].

Symphysiotomy has been a controversial procedure but may well have a role in management of obstructed labour[33]. An important advantage is that women who are suitable for this procedure will not enter future pregnancies with a scar on their uteruses.

Repair of fistulas

There can be no more satisfying surgical procedure in obstetrics and gynaecology than the successful repair of an obstetric fistula. James Marion Sims carried out the first surgical repair in the USA in 1849. There are a number of recent accounts of the techniques for the surgical repair of obstetric fistulas[34]. The illustrated monograph of Waaldijk is particularly good as a practical guide[35]. There remains a need for training of surgeons in some areas of the world in which this dreadful complication of obstructed labour still occurs. Experience in Ethiopia has shown that surgeons do not necessarily need to have medical qualifications.

Conclusions

Obstructed labour remains an important cause of maternal and fetal mortality and morbidity in many parts of the world. Better understanding of the pathophysiology of myometrial contractility in obstructed labour is important—but much can be done at the moment, even with simple clinical facilities, to identify dystocia and to treat it appropriately. Ultimately, the incidence of obstructed labour will be minimized by ensuring adequate nutrition for girls and young women.

References

1   McCarthy M. What's going on at the World Health Organization? *Lancet* 2002; **360**: 1108–10
2   McCarthy M. A brief history of the World Health Organization. *Lancet* 2002; **360**: 1111–2
3   Mahler H. The safe motherhood initiative: a call to action. *Lancet* 1987; **1**: 668–70
4   World Health Organization. *Maternal Mortality Ratios and Rates—A Tabulation of Available Information*, 3rd edn. Geneva: WHO, 1991
5   World Health Organization Maternal Health and Safe Motherhood Programme. World Health Organization partograph in management of labour. *Lancet* 1994; **343**: 1399–404
6   Konje J, Lapido OA. Nutrition and obstructed labour. *Am J Clin Nutr* 2000; **72**: 291S–7S
7   Orach CG. Maternal mortality estimated using the sisterhood method in the Gulu district, Uganda. *Trop Doct* 2000; **30**: 72–4
8   Hoj L, Stensballe J, Aaby P. Maternal mortality in Guinea-Bissau: the use of verbal autopsy in a multi-ethnic population. *Int J Epidemiol* 1999; **28**: 70–6
9   Adanu RM, Obed SA. Ruptured uterus: a seven-year review from Accra, Ghana. *J Obstet Gynaecol Can* 2003; **25**: 225–30
10   Rashmi R, Radhakrishnan G, Vaid NB, Agarwal N. Ruptured uterus—changing Indian scenario. *J Indian Med Assoc* 2001; **99**: 634–7
11   Prual A, Bouvier-Colle MH, de Bernis L, Breart G. Severe maternal morbidity from direct obstetric causes in West Africa: incidence case fatality rates. *Bull World Health Organ* 2000; **78**: 593–602
12   Kelly J, Kwast BE. Epidemiologic study of vesicovaginal fistulas in Ethiopia. *Int Urogynecol J* 1993; **4**: 278–81
13   Wall LL. Fitsari 'dan Duniya. An African (Hausa) praise song about vesicovaginal fistulas. *Obstet Gynecol* 2002; **100**: 1328–32
14   Arrowsmith S, Hamlin EC, Wall LL. Obstructed labor injury complex: obstetric fistula formation and the multifaceted morbidity of maternal birth trauma in the developing world. *Obstet Gynecol Surv* 1996; **51**: 568–74
15   O'Driscoll K, Meagher D. *The Active Management of Labour*. London: WB Saunders, 1980
16   Crowther C, Enkin M, Keirse M, Brown I. Monitoring the progress of labour. In: Chalmers I, Enkin M, Keirse M (eds) *Effective Care in Pregnancy and Childbirth*, vol. II, Oxford: Oxford University Press, 1989
17   Downe S. How average is normality? *Br J Midwifery* 1994; **2**: 303–4
18   Duignan NM, Studd JWW, Hughes AO. Characteristics of normal labour in different racial groups. *Br J Obstet Gynaecol* 1975; **82**: 593–601

19 Friedman EA. Primigravid labor—a graphicostatistical analysis. *Am J Obstet Gynecol* 1955; **6**: 567–89

20 O'Driscoll K, Meagher D, Boylan P. *Active Management of Labour*, 3rd edn. Mosby Year Book Europe Ltd, 1993

21 Friedman EA. Graphic analysis of labor. *Am J Obstet Gynecol* 1954; **68**: 1568–75

22 Walss Rodriguez RJ, Gudino Ruiz F, Tapia Rodriguez S. Labor. Comparative study between Friedman's partogram and conventional descriptive partogram. *Ginecol Obstet Mexico* 1987; **55**: 318–22

23 Philpott RH. Graphic records in labour. *BMJ* 1972; **4**: 163

24 Philpott RH, Castle WM. Cervicographs in the management of labour in primigravidae. *J Obstet Gynaecol Br Cwlth* 1972; **79**: 592–8

25 Lennox CE, Kwast BE. The partograph in community obstetrics. *Trop Doct* 1995; **25**: 56–63

26 Klaus MH, Kennell JH, Robertson SS, Sosa R. Effects of social support during parturition on maternal and infant morbidity. *BMJ* 1986; **2930**: 586–7

27 Hodnett E, Gates S, Hofmeyr GJ, Sakala C. Continuous support for women during childbirth (Cochrane Review). In: *The Cochrane Library, Issue 3, 2003*. Oxford: Update Software

28 Thornton J, Lilford R. Active management of labour: current knowledge and research issues. *BMJ* 1994; **309**: 366–9

29 Olah KA, Gee H. The active mismanagement of labour. *Br J Obstet Gynaecol* 1996; **103**: 729–31

30 Fraser WD, Turcot L, Krauss I, Brisson-Carrol G. Amniotomy for shortening spontaneous labour (Cochrane Review). In: *The Cochrane Library, Issue 3, 2003*. Oxford: Update Software

31 Frigoletto FD, Lieberman E, Lang JM, Cohen A, Barss V, Ringer S, Datta S. A clinical trial of active management of labour. *N Engl J Med* 1995; **333**: 745–50

32 Smaill F, Hofmeyr GJ. Antibiotic prophylaxis for cesarean section (Cochrane Review). In: *The Cochrane Library, Issue 3, 2003*. Oxford: Update Software

33 Bjorklund K. Minimally invasive surgery for obstructed labour: a review of symphysiotomy during the twentieth century (including 5000 cases). *Br J Obstet Gynaecol* 2002; **109**: 236–48

34 Kelly J. Repair of obstetric fistulae. *Obstet Gynaecol* 2002; **4**: 205–11

35 Waaldijk K. *Step-by-step Surgery of Vesicovaginal Fistulas. A Full-color Atlas*. Edinburgh: Campion Press, 1994

Post-partum haemorrhage: definitions, medical and surgical management. A time for change

Hazem El-Refaey* and **Charles Rodeck**[†]

*Chelsea and Westminster Hospital and †Department of Obstetrics and Gynaecology, University College London, London, UK

Any woman who gives birth can have post-partum haemorrhage which may threaten her life. PPH is one of the leading causes of maternal mortality and an important cause for serious morbidity in the developing and developed world. We are at the threshold of major developments in its prevention and treatment due to changing ideas about its definition and medical and surgical management. The implementation of these changes is an essential part of a wider commitment towards saving mothers from complications of childbirth.

Introduction, definitions and classification

Post-partum haemorrhage (PPH) is a clinical problem of indisputable importance to patients, clinicians and to those interested in achieving equity in reproductive health. As a condition it is almost always associated with meaningful implications to patients. Even the mild self-limiting cases have consequences for the patient's puerperium in the form of fatigue, tiredness, failure to breast-feed and possible need for haematinics or blood transfusion. All are symptoms and consequences of anaemia and acute blood loss. The cascade associated with intractable PPH is an entirely different matter however. It is a spiral of events that challenges the acumen of the attending clinicians and their ability to implement the prepared drills of action to handle such a clinical emergency. PPH can transform a normal woman in labour to a critically ill patient within minutes. The management of such a patient is a real test for the thought processes, resources, organizational effort and the education of a labour ward and its staff.

Historically, PPH was one of the leading causes of maternal death in industrialized nations up to the Second World War. It is still a leading cause of maternal death in the rest of the world today. The classification, definition and treatment of PPH have seen almost no change over the

Correspondence to:
Hazem El-Refaey,
Consultant Obstetrician
and Gynaecologist,
Chelsea and Westminster
Hospital,
369 Fulham Road,
London SW10 9NH, UK.
E-mail:
h.elrefaey@imperial.ac.uk

last 50 years. Defined by the World Health Organization (WHO) as post-partum blood loss in excess of 500 ml, it is a clinical diagnosis that encompasses excessive blood loss after delivery of the baby from a variety of sites: uterus, cervix, vagina and perineum[1]. Blood loss during the first 24 h after delivery is known as primary PPH, whereas blood loss from 24 h up to 6 weeks after delivery is termed late or secondary PPH. The bleeding is also classified according to its site. Hence primary PPH is also classified as either placental or extra-placental bleeding.

The definition and classification of PPH have stood the test of time but they are not without problems. For example a cut-off point of 500 ml implies that any loss smaller than this is within normal limits and can therefore be tolerated without risk. This is certainly not the case in countries where severe anaemia is common and where blood loss of as little as 250 ml may constitute a clinical problem[2]. Furthermore, not all placental site bleeding is the same. There is a difference in bleeding from the upper segment to that from the lower segment of the uterus. The bleeding from the former usually if not always responds to uterotonic agents, whereas the latter does not. It is useful to embed this distinction in the literature and in training as it impacts on management options and pathways and on the speed with which they are adopted.

One could argue that the initial administration of uterotonic agents in cases of PPH is nothing more than a clinical test. The outcome of a such test could be positive with cessation of the bleeding. In such a case a retrospective diagnosis of upper segment PPH is made. Continuation of bleeding, on the other hand, would indicate that 'Examination under anaesthesia' to exclude trauma is necessary. If this is excluded and the bleeding continues then this patient might have lower segment bleeding that will require laparotomy to deal with it. B-Lynch sutures or hysterectomy for example might provide the appropriate and curative intervention for cases of lower segment PPH. Wasting time in anticipation of a response to uterotonic agents in these cases will be futile.

The incidence of PPH ranges between 5% and 8% in places where some form of prophylaxis is practised, but may be as high as 18% when a physiological approach is the norm[3]. Physiological control of post-partum bleeding occurs by contraction and retraction of the interlacing myometrial fibres surrounding maternal spiral arteries in the placental bed. Myometrial contraction compresses the spiral arteries and veins, thereby obliterating their lumina. Haemostasis following placental separation is thereby initially a mechanical process not primarily dependent upon an intact coagulation system. Development of this mechanism was a crucial aspect of viviparity without which mammals would not have evolved. However it is flawed: Primary PPH due to uterine atony occurs when the relaxed myometrium fails to constrict these blood vessels, thereby allowing haemorrhage. Since up to one-fifth of maternal cardiac output, which is in excess of 600 ml/min, enters the uteroplacental circulation at term, it is understandable that primary atonic PPH can be catastrophic—capable of exsanguinating the mother within minutes. Whilst uterine atony is responsible for the majority of primary PPH, the surgical obstetrical causes such as injury of the cervix, vagina, paravaginal spaces, perineum and episiotomy comprise about 20% of all primary PPH.

The scale of the problem

The last two decades have witnessed an increasing awareness of gender-related medical problems in the world. Maternal mortality figures have increasingly become an emotive political issue. The lack of improvement in these figures in the developing world reflects the complex nature of the problems these societies face. In some cases calls were made to exert political pressure on governments to tackle the problems. Linking certain aspects of foreign aid to advances in reproductive health was portrayed as an effective leverage to implement change. In some of the cases where improvement was reported it is difficult to ascertain how much of this improvement is a political dressing and how much is a real improvement. The fact remains however that the figures are far too high, reflecting in their distribution the socio-economic divisions around the globe. The exact contribution of PPH to maternal mortality figures is not known precisely because haemorrhage in labour or afterward is usually presented as one group. It is however one of the leading causes of maternal mortality—especially in less developed countries where multi-parity, fibroid uterus and anaemia are common. World-wide it is the most common reason for blood transfusion after delivery and it is esti-mated that at least 150,000 women per annum bleed to death during or immediately after labour. This figure is almost certainly an underestimate. Death due to PPH is reported to represent between 17% and 40% of maternal mortality in some parts of the world[4,5]. Even in developed countries, for example The Netherlands, PPH causes 13% of all recorded maternal deaths. In the USA, it has been reported that obstetric haemor-rhage is responsible for 13% of maternal death with PPH the lethal event in over one-third of these cases[6]. In those parts of the world where blood replacement is not possible due to lack of resources, post-partum severe hypotensive shock leads to considerable morbidity including acute renal failure, partial or total necrosis of the anterior pituitary gland and other organ system injury such as pancreatitis and adult respiratory distress syndrome (ARDS).

To prevent serious morbidity or death from PPH many systems need to be functioning: trained birth attendants, emergency transport systems (the window of time needed to save life is short), availability of blood transfusion and other essential obstetric functions at the first referral level. It is recognized that routine pharmacological use of uterotonic agents is an important prophylactic measure against PPH. Strategies to reduce post-partum bleeding include the use of uterotonic drugs such as oxytocin, Syntometrine (combination of oxytocin and ergometrine) or ergometrine. Other measures include early clamping of the cord and delivery of the placenta by cord traction. These are collectively termed 'active' management of the third stage. With 'passive' (expectant, physiologic, conservative) management, oxytocics are used only if there is excessive bleeding, the cord is clamped relatively late and the placenta delivered with the help of gravity and maternal effort. However, many variations of third stage management exist in which a mixture of active and passive management is used.

Systematic reviews of interventions during the third stage of labour suggest that there are advantages to using active management strategies[7,8]. Prophylactic oxytocics reduce the risk of PPH by about 60% and the need for extra oxytocics by about 70%. Passive management could be practised in low risk women delivering at hospitals or those delivering at home or in clinics who can be transferred to the hospital within a very short time in case of an emergency. This is a likely scenario in industrialized countries. In developing countries, however, there are different factors to consider. In rural areas, access to a skilled birth attendant might not be possible. Transfer to a clinic or hospital in case of an emergency might be slow and complicated. The high incidence of pregnancy anaemia in most developing countries makes it more important to prevent any avoidable blood loss.

The use of Syntometrine however is associated with several problems. Syntometrine possesses hypertensive properties and has been known to produce a rise in blood pressure in women previously known to be normotensive. It is therefore contraindicated in women with hypertension in pregnancy, which may affect about one in seven women[9]. Syntometrine frequently causes nausea and vomiting[7]. Syntometrine and oxytocin have to be given by intramuscular injection requiring a sterile needle and syringe, an important consideration in the developing world in view of the rising incidence of HIV, hepatitis B and C and other blood-borne diseases in many parts of the world. Finally, because oxytocic agents are not stable at high ambient temperatures, they require special storage conditions. When Syntometrine is stored for prolonged periods the temperature must be maintained between 2 and 8°C and it must be protected from light. Studies designed to simulate the storage conditions commonly found in tropical countries found that a variety of brands of ergometrine lost 21–27% of their active ingredients after 1 month, and over 90% after 1 year of storage exposed to light and at 21–25°C[10,11].

These storage requirements are an important barrier to the effective use of oxytocics in the developing world. Oxytocin alone is not without problems although they are not as widely known as those of ergometrine[12–14]. The main preservative used in syntocinon ampoules is chlorobutanol which has a negative effect on cardiac muscle[15,16]. Obstetricians in general are not familiar with its side-effects whilst anaesthetists can easily visualize it on their monitors[17]. Since syntocinon has a direct effect on the heart, it is not allowed to be used intravenously without an infusion in North America. The parenteral nature of syntocinon however is the main obstacle to its wide use around the world.

WHO has what is termed an essential drug list. No uterotonic agent is on this list. The aforementioned problems meant that there is not a suitable one. This omission could only be filled by an agent that, as well as being safe and effective, is also enterally administered, normotensive and thermostable.

Misoprostol and the third stage of labour

Other than oxytocin and ergot preparations, prostaglandins are the only group of drugs that have a potential for routine use in the third stage. Prostaglandin agents are known to possess strong uterotonic features that have been utilized in obstetric practice for three decades. They are widely used for cervical ripening, induction of labour and induction of abortion. They are also known to be useful as a last resort in the management of intractable PPH.

Unlike ergometrine-related agents, prostaglandins are not hypertensive[18]. This, combined with their strong uterotonic effect and apparent superiority in the management of PPH, suggests that they may be the ideal agents for routine prophylactic use in the third stage of labour. To date relatively small controlled trials indicate that injectable prostaglandin analogues seem as effective as Syntometrine[19–22].

The use of misoprostol in Obstetrics and Gynaecology has been nothing short of a revolution in reproductive health care. The therapeutic uses of prostaglandins have become more equitable and new indications and ways of treatment have been pioneered. The wide availability of misoprostol to clinicians and the controversial attitude of the pharmaceutical industry have meant that clinicians have had to take the leadership in its development[23–26]. New regimens and routes of administration were identified and the drug was soon shown to be effective by the oral, vaginal and rectal routes[27,28]. A small study by El-Refaey in 1993 identified the very rapid change in uterine contractility in response to oral and vaginal misoprostol. The study showed that misoprostol administered by these routes is not only absorbed promptly but can also have a considerable impact on uterine contractility in minutes. Figure 1 shows the change in intrauterine pressures in three patients who were pre-treated with mifepristone 36 h earlier. The vertical arrows highlight the point of administering misoprostol whilst the transverse arrows highlight the length of time taken to achieve a change in uterine contractility. This confirmed uterotonic action of misoprostol in early and late pregnancy, led El-Refaey et al[29] later to consider its use in the third stage of labour. The initial report showed promising efficacy and identified shivering as a potential side-effect.

The proposal to use misoprostol to prevent and treat PPH has been investigated in the last 5 years. El-Refaey et al compared misoprostol 500 μg administered before delivery of the placenta to women receiving other standard uterotonic agents in the third stage in a randomized trial of 1000 patients. The rates of PPH and the need for blood transfusion were similar[30]. Surbek et al[31] also conducted a double-blind randomized controlled trial comparing a single oral dose of misoprostol (600 μg) with placebo in the third stage of labour. The 'obstetrician estimated the blood loss' and the difference in haematocrit before and after delivery were measured. The mean estimated blood loss and haematocrit difference were significantly lower in women who received misoprostol than those who received the placebo. Whereas the need for additional oxytocin was lower in the misoprostol group, shivering was more common in the misoprostol arm.

The uterotonic efficacy of misoprostol in the third stage of labour has also been demonstrated by an objective reproducible method, which uses a catheter-tip intrauterine pressure transducer. This tool was used by Chong et al[32] to examine the effect of oral misoprostol in varying doses (200–800 μg) on the post-partum uterus and to compare its uterine contractility pattern to that following intramuscular Syntometrine. The study confirmed that the cumulative uterine activity with all doses of misoprostol and Syntometrine were similar.

The potential of misoprostol as a therapeutic agent for this phase of labour was also recognized by WHO, who went on to conduct an ambitious multi-centre, randomized controlled trial involving nine countries[33]. This trial is probably the largest in the field of third stage of labour and was designed to compare the use of oral misoprostol (600 μg) to 10 IU of oxytocin.

The trial was statistically powered for two primary outcomes: the measured blood loss of 1000 ml or more and the use of additional uterotonic agents, and 20,000 women were recruited. Unfortunately the trial had several problems[34–37]. At the time of data analysis, it was recognized that information on the route of oxytocin administration was not collected. The authors were therefore unable to quantify the proportion of patients who received the oxytocin intravenously or intramuscularly. Furthermore, there was an unexplained statistical heterogeneity between

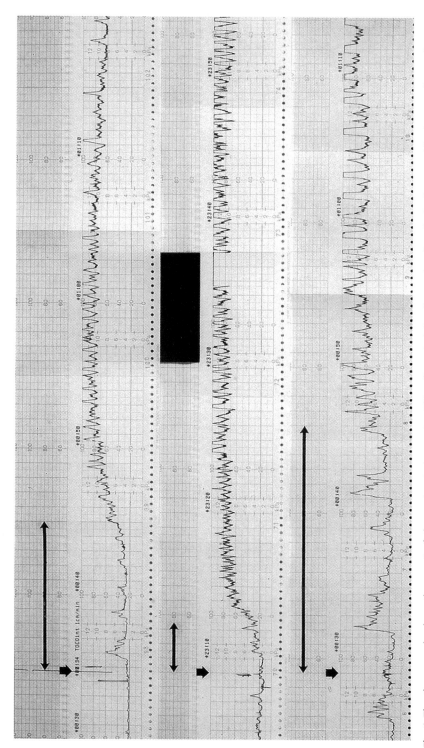

Fig. 1 The three graphs show the onset of change in uterine contractility after administering oral and vaginal misoprostol in three patients who were undergoing medical termination of pregnancy at 9 weeks gestation and were pre-treated with mifepristone 36 h earlier. The top graph is from a patient who received 400 µg misoprostol orally. The middle graph is from a patient who received 800 µg misoprostol orally. The bottom graph is from a patient who received 800 µg misoprostol vaginally. The vertical axis shows the intra-uterine pressure in mmHg. The horizontal axis shows the time in minutes (1 small box = 0.5 min). The vertical arrow indicates the time of the oral administration of misoprostol. The horizontal arrow shows the time interval taken to achieve tetanic uterine contraction after administering misoprostol.

the individual centres for the primary outcome of measured blood loss. Whilst this large trial is often quoted to have shown that there is a 1% difference in PPH between oral misoprostol and oxytocin, the subtle but profound effect of administration of oxytocin by the intravenous route on the results is often overlooked or ignored. This trial also highlighted the limitation of an outcome measure such as measured blood loss in the third stage of labour when it did not correlate with a clinical morbidity marker like 'the need for blood transfusion'. The blood transfusion rate was lower in women in the misoprostol group. However, the WHO trial proved the safety of misoprostol administered orally at doses up to 600 µg.

Pharmacological treatment of post-partum haemorrhage

Ergometrine, and subsequently oxytocin were introduced in the treatment of PPH on the basis of biological and pharmacological principles. The identification of their uterotonic features and the recognition that uterine atony plays a major role in PPH led to their wide adoption as first line drugs in its management. Their prophylactic usage in the third stage of labour was therefore an extension of their role in treatment. It is interesting however that more trial data exist in support of their use in prophylaxis compared to treatment. When the uterotonic features of prostaglandins were later identified they were similarly used in the treatment of PPH. The use of carboprost as an intramyometrial injection, its long list of contraindications and possible side-effects were however prohibitive for the wider use of this prostaglandin analogue. Misoprostol is the most recent drug to be identified as a useful agent in the treatment of PPH and some supporting trial data exist for its use. However, there is a debate about dosage and route of administration.

Misoprostol has been widely investigated by the oral and then the vaginal route for induction of abortion. It soon became clear that the vaginal route is optimal however because the resulting uterine contractility was more potent and side-effects were lower compared to the oral route. Administering misoprostol vaginally however was thought, at least initially, to be unsuitable for management of PPH because of bleeding. The rectal use of misoprostol came as an answer to this problem. The administration of the drug by the rectal or vaginal route might be more practical and effective than the oral route. Inserting the drug vaginally or rectally by the attending clinician is more practical than handling it to a patient who has just given birth to swallow with a glass of water! There are several studies to indicate misoprostol can be used effectively as a preventive measure by the rectal and most recently vaginal routes[38].

O'Brien *et al*[39] reported in a pilot study that misoprostol 1000 µg given rectally is an effective intervention in women with severe PPH, unresponsive to standard uterotonic agents. Subsequent observational studies and a recent randomized study support the use of rectal misoprostol (800 µg) in the treatment of PPH[40]. The latter trial also concluded that misoprostol is more effective than a combination of intramuscular Syntometrine injection and oxytocin infusion. Interestingly, although the oxytocin bolus and infusion is a standard practice in treatment of PPH, there is little research to support the use of this regime[41]. The addition of misoprostol to this therapeutic drill seems to be more supported by scientific data than the use of any of the other uterotonic agents.

The rectal use of misoprostol spread quite quickly based on these clinical studies. Hospital management protocols are changing to include the drug in the guidelines of post-partum management. A recent survey from Norway has shown that 20% of obstetricians now use misoprostol in the treatment of PPH[42]. This is despite the fact that, until recently, no pharmacokinetic study had shown that misoprostol is absorbed from the rectum[43].

Surgical management of intractable post-partum haemorrhage

A patient who fails to respond to uterotonic agents and continues to bleed will quickly become haemodynamically unstable and develop a cascade of clotting abnormalities. The spectre of maternal mortality can then only be prevented by initiating surgical haemostasis sooner rather than later. The nature, timing and extent of these invasive interventions will depend on the sophistication of the health facility which handles this medical crisis. The fate of such a woman will therefore vary widely, depending not only on where she lives in the world but also on where she lives in her own country.

Traditionally, total abdominal hysterectomy provided the ultimate cure. The procedure is technically different from hysterectomy for gynaecological reasons. The main difference is identifying and removing the lower uterine segment. This might be the curative part of the procedure and has to be handled with care. The bladder has to be reflected, dissected and pushed inferiorly and laterally to minimize the chances of bladder injury and ureteric injury. The boundaries of the lower uterine segment are ill-defined and it can be difficult to identify the cervix. Often it can only be partially removed.

Delaying the decision to carry out post-partum hysterectomy can be catastrophic because the patient may deteriorate much further and faster than anticipated so that it becomes impossible later to carry out what could have been a life-saving intervention. Hysterectomy should not be delayed until the patient is in extremes or while less definitive procedures of which the surgeon has little experience are attempted. Performing hysterectomy in a timely fashion is therefore a sign of maturity of the team looking after the patient. The pressures to preserve fertility and avoid a hysterectomy can also be equally great and several techniques have evolved in recent decades. Interventions to occlude the blood supply to the uterus or to tamponade the uterine cavity are options to avoid inevitable hysterectomy.

Ligation of the internal iliac arteries has been used but requires complex dissection of the lateral pelvic wall. Vascular embolization procedures have become established and are less invasive interventions with well documented curative effect. The technique involves inserting a catheter in the femoral artery going into the large circulation and then to the uterine vessels. Embolization at this point will at least lower the blood pressure around the uterus[44]. These techniques require a multidisciplinary approach and trained personnel who might not be available in many district hospitals even in industrialized nations.

Within the last decade there has been renewed interest in new uterine tamponade procedures such as balloon compression and other procedures, e.g. the B-Lynch suture. The oldest form of tamponade, uterine packing, has a long history in obstetrics and was widely used in the management of PPH before prostaglandin agents were an option or because of their expense. A 20-m-long gauze pack has to be tightly inserted inside the uterus. For it to work, it must start at the fundus of the uterus otherwise bleeding will continue above the pack. The success of the procedure is dependent on these points and this may become apparent some hours later. Anxieties about the efficacy of the technique and its potential to act as a focus of infection and to cause pressure necrosis on adjacent organs have led to alternative approaches such as the Sengstaken balloon compression. Arulkumaran and others described 14 cases of intractable PPH who avoided surgery by the use of this balloon[45].

The B-Lynch technique is a suture that envelops and compresses the uterus and was first described[46] in a case series in 1997. Compared to hysterectomy or to vascular embolization, the B-Lynch suture is a much simpler procedure and its technique can be easily mastered. It does not require special training and is illustrated in Figure 2a and b. Experience with this technique is promising but the evidence is limited to case reports.

Conclusion

PPH is an important cause of maternal morbidity. We now have new pharmacological and technical developments for prevention and treatment which can greatly reduce its incidence and sequelae. Wider use

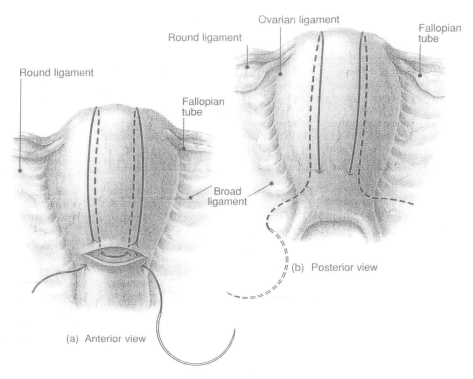

Fig. 2 (a) The anterior view of the uterus showing the application of the B-Lynch suture. (b) The posterior view of the uterus showing the application of the B-Lynch suture.

of thermostable prostaglandins like misoprostol and dissemination of knowledge about new tamponade procedures can minimize its incidence and limit its serious sequelae. The safety of the third stage of labour, and the incidence of PPH and its complications will remain linked however to the wider issues of reproductive health in general and more specifically to the funding and training needed to raise the standard of care offered to women in labour in many parts of the world.

References

1   WHO. *The Prevention and Management of Postpartum Haemorrhage. Report of a Technical Working Group. Geneva 3–6 July 1989*. World Health Organization/Maternal and Child Health 90.7. Geneva: WHO, 1990

2   Lawson JB. Obstetric haemorrhage. In: Lawson JB, Stewart DB (eds) *Obstetrics and Gynaecology in the Tropics*. London: Edward Arnold, 1967; 155–9

3   Prendiville W, Elbourne D. Care during the third stage of labour. In: Chalmers I, Enkin M, Keirse MJNC (eds) *Effective Care in Pregnancy and Childbirth*. Oxford: Oxford University Press, 1989; 1145–69

4   World Health Organization. *Preventing Maternal Deaths*. Geneva: WHO, 1989; 107–36

5   World Health Organization. *Maternal Mortality A Global Factbook*. Geneva: WHO, 1991; 3–16

6   Roberts WE. Emergent obstetric management of postpartum hemorrhage. *Obstet Gynecol Clin North Am* 1995; **22**: 283–302

7   Prendiville WJ, Harding JE, Elbourne DR, Stirrat GM. The Bristol third stage trial: active versus physiological management of third stage of labour. *BMJ* 1988; **297**: 1295–300

8   Prendiville WJ, Elbourne D, McDonald S. Active versus expectant management in the third stage of labour. *Cochrane Database Syst Rev* 2000; **3**: CD000007

9   Sibai BM. Pre-eclampsia-eclampsia. *Curr Probl Obstet Gynecol Fertil* 1990; **13**: 1

10 Walker GJ, Hogerzeil HV. Potency of ergometrine in tropical countries. *Lancet* 1988; **2**: 393

11 Hogerzeil HV, Walker GJ. Instability of (methyl)ergometrine in tropical climates: an overview. *Eur J Obstet Gynecol Reprod Biol* 1996; **69**: 25–9

12 Botting JH, Manley DG. The action of commercial preparations of oxytocin and vasopressin on the smooth muscle of the gut. *J Pharm Pharmacol* 1967; **19**: 66

13 Maycock EJ, Russell WC. Anaphylactoid reaction to Syntocinon. *Anaesth Intens Care* 1993; **21**: 211–2

14 Hofmann H, Goerz G, Plewig G. Anaphylactic shock from chlorobutanol-preserved oxytocin. *Contact Dermatitis* 1986; **15**: 241

15 Rosaeg OP, Cicutti NJ, Labow RS. The effect of oxytocin on the contractile force of human atrial trabeculae. *Anesth Analg* 1998; **86**: 40–4

16 Barrigon S, Tejerina T, Delgado C, Tamargo J. Effects of chlorbutol on 45Ca movements and contractile responses of rat aorta and its relevance to the actions of Syntocinon. *J Pharm Pharmacol* 1984; **36**: 521–6

17 Weis Jr FR, Markello R, Mo B, Bochiechio P. Cardiovascular effects of oxytocin. *Obstet Gynecol* 1975; **46**: 211–4

18 El Refaey H, Templeton A. Early abortion induction by a combination of mifepristone and oral misoprostol: a comparison between two dose regimens of misoprostol and their effect on blood pressure. *Br J Obstet Gynaecol* 1994; **101**: 792–6

19 Abdel-Aleem H, El Nashar I, Abdel-Aleem A. Management of severe postpartum hemorrhage with misoprostol. *Int J Gynaecol Obstet* 2001; **72**: 75–6

20 Poeschmann RP, Doesburg WH, Eskes TK. A randomized comparison of oxytocin, sulprostone and placebo in the management of the third stage of labour. *Br J Obstet Gynaecol* 1991; **98**: 528–30

21 Kerekes L, Domokos N. The effect of prostaglandin F2 alpha on third stage labor. *Prostaglandins* 1979; **18**: 161–6

22 Van Selm M, Kanhai HH, Keirse MJ. Preventing the recurrence of atonic postpartum hemorrhage: a double-blind trial. *Acta Obstet Gynecol Scand* 1995; **74**: 270–4

23 Friedman MA. Manufacturer's warning regarding unapproved uses of misoprostol. *N Engl J Med* 2001; **344**: 61

24 Gebhardt DO. Misoprostol in a topsyturvy world. *J Med Ethics* 2001; **27**: 205

25 Mackenzie WE. Misoprostol and the politics of fear. *Lancet* 2001; **357**: 1296

26 Wagner M. Misoprostol and the politics of convenience. *Lancet* 2001; **357**: 2142

27 Goldberg AB, Greenberg MB, Darney PD. Misoprostol and pregnancy. *N Engl J Med* 2001; **344**: 38–47

28 Mousa HA, Alfirevic Z. Treatment for primary postpartum haemorrhage (Cochrane Review). *Cochrane Database Syst Rev* 2003; **1**: CD003249

29 El Refaey H, O'Brien P, Morafa W, Walder J, Rodeck C. Misoprostol for third stage of labour. *Lancet* 1996; **347**: 1257

30 El Refaey H, Nooh R, O'Brien P, Abdalla M, Geary M, Walder J, Rodeck C. The misoprostol third stage of labour study: a randomised controlled comparison between orally administered misoprostol and standard management. *Br J Obstet Gynaecol* 2000; **107**: 1104–10

31 Surbek DV, Fehr PM, Hosli I, Holzgreve W. Oral misoprostol for third stage of labor: a randomized placebo-controlled trial. *Obstet Gynecol* 1999; **94**: 255–8

32 Chong YS, Chua S, El Refaey H, Choo WL, Chanrachakul B, Tai BC, Rodeck C, Arulkumaran S. Postpartum intrauterine pressure studies of the uterotonic effect of oral misoprostol and intramuscular syntometrine. *Br J Obstet Gynaecol* 2001; **108**: 41–7

33 Gulmezoglu AM, Villar J, Ngoc NT *et al*. WHO multicentre randomised trial of misoprostol in the management of the third stage of labour. *Lancet* 2001; **358**: 689–95

34 El Refaey H. Use of misoprostol in third stage of labour. *Lancet* 2002; **359**: 707–8

35 Khan R, Sharma S. Use of misoprostol in third stage of labour. *Lancet* 2002; **359**: 708–9

36 O'Brien P, Lokugamage AU, Guillebaud J, Rodeck CH. Use of misoprostol in third stage of labour. *Lancet* 2002; **359**: 708–10

37 Shannon C, Winikoff B. Use of misoprostol in third stage of labour. *Lancet* 2002; **359**: 709–10

38 Quiroga DR, Esparza AM, Batiza RV, Coronado LO, Hernandez AS, Martinez CJ. [In Process Citation]. *Ginecol Obstet Mex* 2002; **70**: 572–5

39 O'Brien P, El Refaey H, Gordon A, Geary M, Rodeck CH. Rectally administered misoprostol for the treatment of postpartum hemorrhage unresponsive to oxytocin and ergometrine: a descriptive study. *Obstet Gynecol* 1998; **92**: 212–4

40 Lokugamage AU, Sullivan KR, Niculescu I *et al*. A randomized study comparing rectally administered misoprostol versus Syntometrine combined with an oxytocin infusion for the cessation of primary post partum hemorrhage. *Acta Obstet Gynecol Scand* 2001; **80**: 835–9

41 Daro AF, Gollin HA, Lavieri V. Management of postpartum hemorrhage by prolonged administration of oxytocics. *Am J Obstet Gynecol* 1952; **64**: 1163–4

42 Bjornerem A, Acharya G, Oian P, Maltau JM. Post partum haemorrhage. Prophylaxis and treatment in Norway. *Tidsskr Nor Laegeforen* 2002; **122**: 2536–7

43 Khan R, El Refaey H. Pharmacokinetics and adverse effect profile of rectally administered misoprostol in the third stage of labour. *Obstet Gynecol* 2003; **101**: 968–74

44 Corr P. Arterial embolization for haemorrhage in the obstetric patient. *Best Pract Res Clin Obstet Gynaecol* 2001; **15**: 557–61

45 Condous G, Arulkumaran S, Symonds I *et al*. The tamponade test in the management of massive post partum haemorrhage. *Obstet Gynecol* 2003; **101**: 767–71

46 B-Lynch C, Coker A, Lawal AH, Abu J, Cowen MJ. The B-Lynch surgical technique for the control of massive post partum haemorrhage: an alternative to hysterectomy? Five cases reported. *Br J Obstet Gynaecol* 1997; **104**: 372–5

Perinatal psychiatric disorders: a leading cause of maternal morbidity and mortality

Margaret Oates

Nottingham University Medical School, Nottingham, UK

The Confidential Enquiry into Maternal Deaths 1997 to 1999 finds that psychiatric disorder, and suicide in particular, is the leading cause of maternal death. Suicide accounted for 28% of maternal deaths. Women also died from other complications of psychiatric disorder and a significant minority from substance misuse. Some of the findings of the Confidential Enquiry confirm long established knowledge about postpartum psychiatric disorder. The findings highlight the severity and early onset of serious postpartum mental illness and of the risk of recurrence following childbirth faced by women with a previous history of serious mental illness either following childbirth or at other times. These findings led to the recommendation that all women should be asked early in their pregnancy about a previous history of serious psychiatric disorder and that management plans should be in place with regard to the high risk of recurrence following delivery. Other findings of the Enquiry were new and challenged some of the accepted wisdoms of obstetrics and psychiatry. It is likely that the suicide rate following delivery is not significantly different to other times in women's lives and for the first 42 days following delivery may be elevated. This calls into question the so-called 'protective effect of maternity'. The overwhelming majority of the suicides died violently, contrasting with the usual finding that women are more likely to die from an overdose of medication. Compared to other causes of maternal death, the suicides were older and socially advantaged. The Enquiry findings suggest that the risk profile for women at risk of suicide following delivery may be different to that in women at other times and in men. None of the women who died had been admitted at any time to a Mother and Baby Unit and their psychiatric care had been undertaken by General Adult Services. None of the women who died had had a previous episode correctly identified and none had had adequate plans for their proactive care. The conclusion is that there is a need for both Psychiatry and Obstetrics to acknowledge the substantial risk that women with a previous psychiatric history of serious mental illness face following delivery.

Correspondence to:
Dr Margaret Oakes,
Nottingham University
Medical School, Division
of Psychiatry, Duncan
Macmillan House,
Porchester Road,
Nottingham
NG3 6AA, UK.
E-mail: Margaret.Oates@
nottingham.ac.uk

Background

Since antiquity, it has been recognized that some women develop a particularly florid and severe mental illness in the days and weeks following childbirth. Puerperal insanity was first described in the psychiatric literature by Esquirol and later by his pupil Marcé in 1857. Over the last 40 years the epidemiology of this condition, now known as puerperal psychosis, and its clinical features have been well established. The incidence of two per thousand deliveries seems to have been remarkably constant over time[1]. It is also well established that this condition has a tendency to recur following future childbirth[1-3]. Most studies regard puerperal psychosis as a variant of severe affective disorder (manic depressive illness or bipolar disorder)[3]. However this does not do justice to the condition's phenomena, lability and complexity. First rank symptoms of schizophrenia are often present and may result in the categorization of the illness as 'schizo-affective disorder'. A previous history or family history of bipolar disorder substantially increases the risk of developing a puerperal psychosis. Some women may go on not only to have postpartum episodes but non-postpartum episodes as well. This further supports the view that puerperal psychosis belongs to the spectrum of affective disorders[3].

Puerperal psychosis remains a rare event. Since the 1960s there has been increasing research and clinical interest in the more common non-psychotic affective disorders that follow childbirth, now known as post-natal depression or its acronym 'PND'. In total, 10–13% of women are said to suffer from a postnatal depressive illness that meets the criteria for DCM IIIR minor and major depression[4]. These illnesses will include a variety of subtypes and severities as at other times. Between 3 and 5% of women will suffer from a moderate to severe depressive illness following childbirth[5]. In addition to the two per thousand women who are admitted to hospital suffering from puerperal psychosis, a further two per thousand will be admitted suffering from non-psychotic illnesses, usually very severe postnatal depression.

The incidence of postpartum psychiatric disorder is shown in Table 1.

The majority of women who develop severe mental illness following childbirth will have been well during pregnancy and previously. However the prevalence of all psychiatric conditions (with a possible exception of anorexia nervosa) is the same at conception as at other times. Few psychiatric disorders are associated with a reduction in biological fertility.

Table 1 Incidence of perinatal psychiatric disorders

15%	'Depression'
10%	PND
3–5%	Moderate/severe depressive illness
2%	Referred psychiatry
0.4%	Admitted
0.2%	Admitted psychosis
0.2%	Births to schizophrenic mothers

Pre-existing psychiatric disorder therefore can complicate pregnancy. Whilst the incidence of serious mental illness in pregnancy is probably lower than at other times[1], depression and anxiety are common in pregnancy and may continue after delivery.

Risk and childbirth

The risk of a woman developing a psychotic episode in the year following delivery is said to be a 14-fold increase in relative risk and for 30 days following the first childbirth a 35-fold increase in risk[1]. The incidence of severe depressive illness and the rate of referral to Psychiatric Services is also increased following childbirth and has been estimated to be at least five times greater than in non-childbearing women[6]. Women with a previous history of bipolar illness or puerperal psychosis face an elevated risk of recurrence following delivery, recently estimated to be as high as one in two[2]. Women with chronic schizophrenia who continue to take their medication throughout pregnancy may not be at elevated risk of a relapse in their condition following delivery[1]. However those who suffer from episodic or paranoid schizophrenia may be at equivalent risk to those who suffer from bipolar disorder[1,7].

Postnatal depression is the commonest postpartum psychiatric disorder. Except for its most severe forms, there is no evidence to suggest that depression is any more common following childbirth than at other times in young women's lives, that is to say women are not at increased risk of suffering from a mild depressive illness following childbirth[4]. However those who have already suffered from postnatal depressive illness, of any severity, following a previous childbirth are at increased risk following subsequent childbirths, a risk estimated at one in three[8].

Perinatal psychiatric disorder can therefore be seen to complicate a substantial number, at least 15%, of maternities both in pregnancy and the postpartum period. A minority of these illnesses will be very severe with risk factors that have a high predictive value and will require specialist care.

The findings of the Confidential Enquiries into Maternal Deaths (CEMD) 1997 to 1999 'Why Mothers Die'[9] reflect established knowledge of serious mental illness following childbirth: the importance of past history and the risk of recurrence as well as the particular severity of serious postpartum illness. However they also reveal new findings which challenge some of the conventional wisdoms of obstetric and psychiatric practice, particularly that suicide is the leading cause of maternal death.

The Confidential Enquiries into Maternal Deaths: psychiatric causes of death

Suicide and other psychiatric deaths have always been reported to the CEMD. However it is only in the last two triennia that a psychiatrist has been a member of the CEMD, and psychiatric deaths separately analysed.

A psychiatric maternal death is one that would not have occurred in the absence of a psychiatric disorder. All psychiatric deaths are classified as indirect or coincidental. An argument could be made for regarding suicide in a woman suffering from puerperal psychosis or severe postnatal depression as a direct death. However it is by no means widely accepted that such illnesses are directly caused by childbirth and neither the ICD 10 nor DCM IV recognize these as specific disorders. The majority of psychiatric deaths were due to suicide, a minority to substance misuse (mainly accidental overdoses of heroin and a few to other causes, for example pulmonary embolism and homicide) (Table 2).

Suicide

Between 1997 and 1999, there were 2,123,614 maternities and 242 maternal deaths, from both direct and indirect causes, reported to the CEMD, a maternal mortality rate of 11.4 per hundred thousand. Adding coincidental and late deaths, the total was 378 maternal deaths, an overall maternal mortality rate of 17.8 per hundred thousand (Table 3).

In total, 11% of the maternal deaths reported to the CEMD were due to psychiatric causes. The majority of the coincidental psychiatric deaths were due to accidental overdose of heroin and 12% of indirect deaths were due to suicide. Thus in cases reported to the CEMD, suicide was the lead cause of indirect death and the second lead cause of death overall (Table 4).

Table 2 Causes of death, Confidential Enquiries into Maternal Death, 1997–99

	Pregnant	Early	Late	Total
Suicide	6	6	16	28
Illicit drugs—overdose	2	0	6	8
Other				6
Pulmonary embolus		1	1	
Adverse drug reactions		1		
Murder		1		
Alcohol-related	2			
Total	10	9	23	42

Table 3 CEMD/UK 1997/99; maternal mortality

2,124,000	Maternities
242 deaths	(direct and indirect)
Mortality	11.4/100,000
Direct	5.0/100,000 falling
Indirect	6.4/100,000 rising
378 deaths total (+ coincidental)	17.8/100,000

Table 4 Suicide leading cause of maternal death; CEMD UK 1997/99

Total psychiatric maternal deaths	
42/378	11%
CEMD suicides	
28/242	12%
Additional 40 'ONS' suicides	
68/242	28%

The ONS Linkage Study

Under ascertainment has been a problem for all Committees of Enquiry and for all suicide research. It was likely that many cases of suicide were not reported to the CEMD, particularly if late in the postpartum year. An Office of National Statistics (ONS) Linkage Study was conducted to complement the 1997/99 CEMD. By linking death certificates with birth certificates in the preceding year, a further 200 maternal deaths were identified, of which 59 were psychiatric. These 59 'extra' deaths included 40 suicides, 8 open verdicts and 11 accidental overdoses of illicit drugs, which were not reported to the CEMD. None of the suicides occurred in the first 42 days after birth. The majority of the 'extra' psychiatric deaths were late indirect or coincidental. The mode of death was known but no other psychiatric information was available for analysis. Adding the 40 suicides to the CEMD data, 28% of maternal deaths were due to suicide, which then emerges as the leading cause of maternal death (Table 4).

The characteristics of maternal suicide

In keeping with the findings of the 1994/1996 CEMD[10], 86% of the suicides died violently, mainly by hanging or jumping. Only three women died from an overdose of medication. Despite the inability to include the ONS cases in this report, the method of suicide was known and the findings of the CEMD in this respect would not have been altered by their inclusion. Previous suicide research has consistently found gender differences in methods of suicide. Women are less likely to die violently and more likely to die from an overdose[11,12].

The findings of both the CEMD and the ONS Linkage Study stand in stark contrast to this.

Compared to maternal deaths from physical causes and from substance misuse, maternal suicides were distinguished by being relatively socially advantaged and supported. The majority had higher education and a worrying number were health professionals. This confirms recent suicide research[13] which finds that female suicide is less associated with unemployment, adversity, single status and divorce than is male suicide.

The protective effect of maternity?

The suicide rate in women is lower than in men, decreasing at a greater rate and thought to be lowest of all in pregnancy and the 2 years following the birth[11,13,14], leading to the widespread belief in the 'protective effect of maternity'. The suicide rate amongst all women is estimated to be 3.4 per hundred thousand[12].

The incidence of postpartum mental illness, admission to psychiatric hospital following delivery and contact rate with Psychiatric Services is well established[1,6]. It is therefore possible to estimate the number of maternities likely to have suffered from puerperal psychosis, to have been in contact with Psychiatric Services or admitted to a psychiatric hospital during 1997–1999.

It can be seen from Table 5 that following delivery, the maternal suicide rate is not significantly different to that of the female suicide rate overall. It can also be seen that the suicide rate in women in contact with Psychiatric Services and in particular those suffering from puerperal psychosis is grossly elevated. These findings must challenge the previously held belief that pregnancy and the postpartum year exerted a protective effect on maternal suicide.

The importance of current and past serious mental illness

In total, 56% of all psychiatric deaths reported to the CEMD and 68% of suicides suffered from a serious mental illness (psychosis or a severe depressive illness). Unfortunately, no diagnosis was possible for the ONS Linkage cases, therefore the finding that the majority of the

Table 5 Maternal suicide. Protective effect of maternity?

- Postpartum:pregnant, 4:1

- Estimated 2 suicides/1000 puerperal psychoses
  Estimated 1 suicide/1000 admissions
  Estimated 0.3 suicides/1000 contacts

- Maternal suicide, 3/100,000 births

- Female suicide, 3.4/100,000 population

women who died from suicide were seriously ill may not be maintained if these missing cases had been included. Nonetheless, all the early suicides were suffering from a serious mental illness and there were no early deaths in the ONS study. All of the early psychiatric deaths had an abrupt onset psychotic illness usually within days of childbirth.

In total, 46% of suicides reported to the CEMD had been admitted to a psychiatric hospital during a previous episode of illness. All of these who died from substance misuse had previous contact with Substance Misuse Services. Of the women with a previous psychiatric history, half had been admitted to a psychiatric hospital following a previous childbirth. This is in keeping with our knowledge of postpartum illness and the known risk of recurrence following childbirth of a previous illness postpartum, or otherwise, of one in two.

There were very few cases where either the Psychiatry or Maternity Services had been aware of the past history and risk of recurrence following delivery and even fewer where management plans had been put in place. Despite the established risk of recurrence following childbirth and despite the clinical knowledge that such illnesses are likely to recur at the same time and in the same way as previously, reports to the coroner suggest that the outcome took all by surprise.

Almost half of the women who died from suicide therefore might not have died if their past history had been accurately identified and if plans for proactive management had been put in place. At the very least they should have received close surveillance for the maximum period at risk following delivery and perhaps prophylactic medication.

Problems with the term 'PND'

The CEMD was surprised to find that in those few cases where a previous postpartum psychiatric history had been recorded in the maternity notes, it was described as postnatal depression (PND) not as a psychosis requiring inpatient treatment. The CEMD speculates that this might have diminished the seriousness of the condition and its need for proactive management. This highlights the importance of not using the term postnatal depression or 'PND' as a generic term for all types of mental illness with an assumption of psychosocial aetiology and management.

Detection or management?

In total, 85% of all the women who died had been identified and were receiving treatment; 46% of the suicides were in contact with Psychiatric

Table 6 CEMD 1997–99; current psychiatric contact

Highest level of psychiatric care provided	Index maternity
Inpatient	9
Outpatient/community mental health team	9
Referral but not seen	4
General practitioner treatment only	6
Substance misuse service	5
No contact	3
Unknown	3

Services, of whom half had been inpatients during the index episode. The majority of those who died from substance misuse had been in contact with Substance Misuse Services during this pregnancy. In only three cases were women not receiving any care (Table 6).

Use of specialist services

None of the women who died from suicide had been seen by a Specialist Perinatal Community Mental Health Team and none of the women who had been admitted, either during the index pregnancy or previously following childbirth, had ever been admitted to a Mother and Baby Unit. All of the women who had been admitted to a psychiatric hospital following childbirth either currently or in the past had therefore been separated from their babies. The impact this had on their management and suicide risk can only be imagined.

Over the last 10 years, initiatives to identify women suffering from postnatal depression in the community have become widespread in the UK. These have mainly involved midwives and health visitors by increasing their awareness of postnatal depression and by the widespread use of screening tools such as the Edinburgh Postnatal Depression Scale (EPDS)[15]. Despite its widespread use, the NICE National Screening Committee[16] does not support the routine use of the EPDS either to predict or to detect postnatal depression[15]. The identification of postnatal depression and the development of treatment protocols in primary care is part of the National Service Framework for Mental Health[17]. By implication, the problem of postpartum mental illness is seen as one to be managed in primary care. There has been much less national emphasis on service provision for those suffering from serious mental illness in relation to childbirth. There are very few specialist Mother and Baby Units in the UK and even fewer Trusts that provide Specialist Liaison Psychiatry Services to Maternity Units[18]. The findings of the CEMD confirm this.

Table 7 Recommendations

- Enquiries about previous psychiatric history, its severity, care received and clinical presentation should be routinely made in a systematic and sensitive way at the antenatal booking clinic

- Protocols for the management of women who are at risk of a relapse or recurrence of a serious mental illness following delivery should be in place in every Trust providing maternity services

- The use of the term post nataldepression or PND should not be used as a generic term for all types of psychiatric disorder. Details of previous illness should be sought and recorded in line with the recommendations above

- Women who have a past history of serious psychiatric disorder, postpartum or non-postpartum, should be assessed by a psychiatrist in the antenatal period and a management plan instituted with regard to the high risk of recurrence following delivery

- Women who have suffered from serious mental illness either following childbirth or at other times should be counselled about the possible recurrence of that illness following further pregnancies

CEMD recommendations

Recommendations informed by the key findings of the enquiries are shown in Table 7. They are included in the clinical risk management standards for Maternity Services issued by the Clinical Negligence Scheme for Trusts[19]. It is of concern that in many localities the skills and resources to meet these standards may not be in place. Similar recommendations have been made in the past by the Royal College of Psychiatrists[18] and the Framework for Maternity Services in Scotland[20].

Conclusions

Suicide following childbirth is rare but the rates are higher than previously thought. Suicide is the leading cause of maternal death. Psychiatric morbidity is common during pregnancy and in the postpartum period. Much is severe and some predictable and preventable.

Some women died despite exemplary care. For others it is impossible to know, because of the methodology of the CEMD, whether factors that appear to have contributed to their deaths were not also to be found in women who did not die. Nonetheless a quarter of suicides might not have died if their high risk of postpartum recurrence had been identified and managed.

The findings, that suicide is now the leading cause of maternal death and that the profile of women who kill themselves following delivery is different to that of other women and men, are new. They will hopefully inform Psychiatric Practice, particularly in regard to risk assessment.

The finding that a previous psychiatric history, postpartum or otherwise, predicts a high rate of recurrence following delivery is not new. It is consistent with research findings over the last 40 years. That these should have had apparently such little impact on psychiatric and obstetric practice is concerning. Unique amongst the known antecedents of psychiatric illness, childbirth comes with a 9 month warning, ample time for the detection of risk and putting into place of management plans. Half of the women who died following delivery were suffering from serious mental illness. For half of these women, their deaths might have been prevented if systems had been in place for the identification of their previous psychiatric history at booking and protocols had been in place for the management of their postpartum period. For others, better management of their acute postpartum illness might have improved the outcome. Hopefully the findings too will inform psychiatric and obstetric practice.

The suggestion that the widespread acceptance of postnatal depression 'PND' might have been counter-productive for those suffering from severe mental illness was unexpected. It perhaps leads to the conclusion that differential diagnosis is as important in perinatal psychiatry as it is in other specialities of medicine.

Hopefully, the recommendations of the CEMD will save the lives of some women in the future. They should also improve the care of the majority of women with serious mental illness associated with childbirth.

References

1 Kendell RE, Chalmers KC, Platz C. Epidemiology of puerperal psychoses. *Br J Psychiatry* 1987; **150**: 662–73

2 Wieck A, Kumar R, Hirst AD, Marks NM, Campbell IC, Checkley SA. Increased sensitivity of dopamine receptors and recurrence of affective psychosis after childbirth. *BMJ* 1991; **303**: 613–6

3 Dean C, Williams RJ, Brockington IF. Is puerperal psychosis the same as bipolar manic-depressive disorder? A family study. *Psychol Med* 1989; **19**: 637–47

4 O'Hara MW, Swain AM. Rates & risk of post partum depression—a meta-analysis. *Int Rev Psychiatry* 1996; **8**: 37–54

5 Cox J, Murray D, Chapman G. A controlled study of the onset prevalence and duration of postnatal depression. *Br J Psychiatry* 1993; **163**: 27–41

6 Oates M. Psychiatric Services for women following childbirth. *Int Rev Psychiatry* 1996; **8**: 87–98

7 Davies A, McIvor RJ, Kumar C. Impact of childbirth on a series of schizophrenic mothers. *Schizophr Res* 1995; **16**: 25–31

8 Cooper P, Murray L. The course and recurrence of postnatal depression: evidence for the specificity of the diagnostic concept. *Br J Psychiatry* 1995; **166**: 191–5

9 National Institute for Clinical Excellence. *Why Mothers Die 1997–1999. The Confidential Enquiries into Maternal Deaths in the United Kingdom (CEMD)*. London: RCOG Press, 2001

10 Department of Health. Deaths from psychiatric causes, suicide and substance abuse. In *Why Mothers Die. Report on Confidential Enquiries into Maternal Deaths in the United Kingdom 1994–1996*. London: Her Majesty's Stationery Office, 1998

11 Hawton K. Sex and suicide: Gender differences in suicidal behaviour. *Br J Psychiatry* 2000; **177**: 484–5

12 Schapira K, Linsley KR, Linsley JA, Kelly TP, Kay DK. Relationship of suicide rates to social factors and availability of lethal methods. *Br J Psychiatry* 2001; **178**: 458–64

13 Qin P, Agerbo E, Westergard-Nielsen N, Eriksson T, Mortensen PO. Gender differences in risk factors for suicide. *Br J Psychiatry* 2000; **177**: 546–50

14   Appleby L. Suicidal behaviour in childbearing women. *Int Rev Psychiatry* 1996; **8**: 107–15
15   Cox JL, Holden JM, Sagovsky R. Detection of postnatal depression: development of the 10-item Edinburgh Postnatal Depression Scale (EPDS). *Br J Psychiatry* 1987; **150**: 782–6
16   National Screening Committee. *Screening for Postnatal Depression*. London: Department of Health, 2001
17   Department of Health. *The National Service Framework for Mental Health. Modern Standards and Service Models*. London: Department of Health, 1999
18   Royal College of Psychiatrists. *CR88. Perinatal Mental Health Services. Recommendations for Provision of Services for Childbearing Women*. London: Royal College of Psychiatrists, 2001
19   Clinical Negligence Scheme for Trusts. *Clinical Risk Management Standards for Maternity Services 2002*. NHS Litigation Authority, 2002
20   Scottish Executive. *Framework for Maternity Services I Scotland*. Edinburgh: NHS Scotland, 2001

Near misses: a useful adjunct to maternal death enquiries

RC Pattinson* and **M Hall†**

MRC Maternal and Infant Health Care Strategies Research Unit, University of Pretoria, South Africa and †Department of Obstetrics & Gynaecology, Aberdeen Maternity Hospital, Aberdeen, UK

In developed countries where maternal death is rare, the factors surrounding the death are often peculiar to the event and are not generalizable, making analysis of maternal deaths less useful. *Near misses* are defined as pregnant women with severe life-threatening conditions who nearly die but, with good luck or good care, survive. Incorporation of *near misses* into maternal death enquiries would strengthen these audits by allowing for more rapid reporting, more robust conclusions, comparisons to be made with maternal deaths, reinforcing lessons learnt, establishing requirements for intensive care and calculating comparative indices. The survival of a pregnant woman is dependent on the disease, her basic health, the health care facilities and personnel of the health care system. The criteria currently used to identify a *near miss* vary greatly. However, areas with similar health care facilities, medical records and personnel should be able to agree on suitable criteria, making their incorporation into maternal death enquiries feasible.

Introduction

Correspondence to:
RC Pattinson, Department of Obstetrics and Gynaecology, Kalafong Hospital, Private Bag X396, Pretoria 0001, South Africa. E-mail: rcpattin@kalafong.up.ac.za

An outcome-audit is a retrospective analysis of events that were associated with the particular outcome. To be of use, the outcome must be important, clearly defined and occur frequently enough so that the information gained will be useful for the population studied.

Confidential enquiries into maternal deaths are a common and useful outcome-audit. Obviously death is a very clear end point, making identification and collection of cases simple provided that the death occurs in a health facility. In circumstances where maternal death is or has been fairly frequent, the common causes of maternal death and the modifiable factors associated with the death have been identified. This has served as a diagnostic tool for identifying problems within the health care system and allowed for modification of the system. Confidential enquiries into maternal deaths have been associated with a fall in maternal mortality ratios, clearly documented in the UK[1] over 50 years. The exact causes of the fall in death ratios are not of course known but the Enquiry Reports and their recommendations are thought to have contributed.

However, maternal deaths in developed countries are now rare, and the factors that surround the death are often peculiar to the event, complex and are not generalizable. This does not mean that pregnancy is a safe condition in developed countries. Waterstone et al[2] reported a severe obstetric morbidity rate of 12.0 per 1000 births, and a 'severe morbidity to mortality' ratio of 118:1 in the South East Thames region. Contrary to what would be expected, the common causes of maternal mortality are not the same as the common causes of maternal morbidity. The two most common causes of severe morbidity were severe haemorrhage at 6.7 per 1000 births and complications of hypertension in pregnancy at 4.6 per 1000 deliveries in the London area[2]. However, in the confidential enquiry into maternal deaths in the UK for 1997–1999[3], there were only seven deaths due to haemorrhage and 15 deaths due to complications of hypertension but 35 deaths due to thrombosis and thromboembolism and 35 due to cardiac disease. This is due to the success that modern medicine has had in treating some previously fatal conditions. The diseases causing death are often very rare and information gained from analysing the death is, although useful, limited to those very few people with the condition. For example, congenital heart disease is an important contributor to maternal death in the UK, but congenital heart disease is a rare condition[4].

If an outcome-audit in a developed country is to be conducted as a method of assessing the quality of maternal care, a more appropriate outcome other than death needs to be defined. Prevention of maternal mortality is obviously the aim of obstetricians; hence an outcome-audit of severe acute maternal morbidity would be a useful adjunct to an assessment of maternal deaths, and would concentrate on the management of morbidity once it has occurred. Prevention of maternal morbidity would require data on the population incidence of conditions such as pre-eclampsia and criterion-based audit of the management of a sample of cases.

In the developed world, where very few births occur out of hospital, and can be included in the analysis as civil registration is comprehensive, it may be possible to study inter-regional and secular change in rates of severe morbidity either per maternity, or per case of a given complication. For example, the incidence of status epilepticus per case of epilepsy might be used as an index of how good was ante- and intrapartum care. The situation is more complex for pre-eclampsia, which, because it is a multisystem disorder, might result in eclampsia, a cerebrovascular event, renal failure, or pulmonary oedema. Rates of pulmonary oedema might be used as a measure of the quality of fluid management in acute cases.

It is however difficult to analyse data on prevention of severe maternal morbidity in developing countries because obstetric complications and consequent severe morbidity may present in the community setting and may or may not be referred to seek care in hospitals. Improvements in the system of care that result in more such referrals should, provided that care is of high quality, prevent severe morbidity and indeed mortality, but may appear to increase severe morbidity if referrals are late in the course of disease. Information about events in the community is essential for sensible interpretation of changes.

Definition of maternal morbidity

The definition of severe maternal morbidity is crucial to establishing an audit of maternal morbidity. It must comply with the previously mentioned prerequisites, namely be easily definable, important and occur frequently enough. The World Health Organization (WHO) defines direct obstetric morbidity[5] as resulting from obstetric complications of the pregnancy states (pregnancy, labour and puerperium) from interventions, omissions, incorrect treatment, or from a chain of events resulting from any of the above. The definition is clearly linked to the health care system and implies that all morbidity is preventable, which is obviously not true. Developing an audit system based on this definition is not advisable, though the analysis of the management of cases could follow this pattern.

All health care workers must intuitively understand the definition used, even if the criteria by which such a case is identified are not. A high threshold for defining morbidity would be useful; otherwise the number of cases generated will overwhelm the system. A high threshold would make a comparison with maternal deaths more relevant. For this reason, the term *near miss* has been borrowed from the airline industry. It should be noted that its use in the context of maternity care is quite different to its use in air traffic control[6] where a process has occurred and two aircraft pass too closely to each other but an accident is avoided. This would be analogous to identification by routine audit of prescription errors in the labour ward that may or may not cause a clinical problem. Here we are discussing an *outcome* audit. There are various definitions of *near miss*, all of which express the same thing:

1   A severe life-threatening obstetric complication necessitating an urgent medical intervention in order to prevent likely death of the mother[7].

2   Any pregnant or recently delivered woman, in whom immediate survival is threatened and who survives by chance or because of the hospital care she received[8].

3   A very ill woman who would have died had it not been that luck and good care was on her side[9].

Having a clear understanding of what a *near miss* is, however, does not lead to uniformity in defining the criteria by which a case is identified. How much blood must be lost before a pregnant woman is nearly dead, 1.5 or 2.5 litres? The criteria that have been used to define this life-threatening event have been very different. This is partly due to the context in which the *near miss* occurred. The general state of health of the woman and the health facilities available to her determine the chance of her dying. A woman with prior anaemia may die with a relatively small loss. The facilities available will also determine what care can be given, for example if no blood is available then a blood transfusion cannot be given. The definition used in an environment where intensive care facilities are not available will obviously not include admission to intensive care as a criterion. For this area of morbidity, the *near miss* rate, and the mortality index, will be determined by the threshold chosen.

The search for a universally acceptable set of criteria is not attainable, although the conceptual definition of a *near miss* is. The criteria selected must be locally usable and relevant[10]. They need to be locally generated and consensus attained in their choice. For example it should be possible for developed countries to develop criteria that would be universally acceptable to the whole country because the level of the facilities available is more or less the same. They have intensive care monitoring and treatment facilities on which criteria can be based. The larger the area that uses the criteria, the more valuable the audit will be in comparing different sites and gaining relevant information for that area. Developing countries have a much larger problem in attaining consensus, because of the lack of intensive care monitoring and treatment facilities. If death rates are high, maternal death audits would be a priority but in a feasibility study carried out in four countries, some harmonization of *near miss* audits was possible[10].

There are essentially three methods of identifying severe maternal morbidity: by defining clinical criteria related to a specific disease entity such as pre-eclampsia; a specific intervention such as admission to an intensive care unit or procedure such as a hysterectomy or massive blood transfusion; or a method whereby organ system dysfunction is defined.

Clinical criteria related to a specific disease entity

This was the route taken by Waterstone *et al*[2]. They carefully defined disease-specific morbidities, namely severe pre-eclampsia, eclampsia, HELLP syndrome, severe haemorrhage, severe sepsis and uterine rupture. Using this system, they recorded an incidence of severe maternal morbidity of 12 per 1000 births. The criteria used, while clearly indicating maternal morbidity, have too low a threshold of morbidity to be called *near misses*. Furthermore, the most common direct cause of maternal mortality was omitted, namely pulmonary embolus, because of the difficulty of diagnosing pulmonary emboli accurately when they are not fatal. This illustrates part of the problem of a system based on a specific disease entity. The system also left out early pregnancy complications such as ectopic pregnancies and abortions.

The system has various advantages in that it is straightforward to interpret, data can be obtained retrospectively from case notes or registers and the quality of care of that particular disease can be assessed. However, the London study was a research study and could not be carried out routinely without major expenditure.

The ability to examine the quality of care of a specific disease entity had been well illustrated by Bouvier-Colle *et al*[11]. Cases of severe obstetric haemorrhage were analysed to determine what factors related to health services in France might explain substandard care. Severe obstetric haemorrhage was defined as a haemorrhage occurring at the time of pregnancy outcome if blood loss equalled 1.5 litres, required plasma expanders, equalled 2.5 litres over 24 h or the equivalent expressed in packed cells, or resulted in transfusion, hysterectomy or maternal death. The cases were retrospectively identified and data collected by trained investigators. Criteria for quality of care were selected based on the international literature or because the expert group considered them to be essential. Importantly, 23% of the cases could not be assessed due to poor documentation. However the group found that lack of a 24-h on-site anaesthetist at the hospital and low volume of deliveries were the factors associated with substandard care. This study identified the need for the reorganization of obstetric services in the three French regions, and clearly illustrates the value of this type of audit.

Intervention-based criteria

In most developed countries, admission to an intensive care unit or the requirement of critical care have been used as the criteria to identify *near misses*[12-14]. This system has the advantage that it is simple to identify the cases. However, there are major disadvantages. The most obvious problem is the accessibility of intensive care beds for patients requiring them. In the UK, only 31% of the maternal deaths were recorded as having intensive care[15] possibly because most maternity units have high dependency care available. The major reasons for lack of admission to intensive care were that the death occurred before admission, the lack of availability of beds or because of the distance between the maternity unit and intensive care facilities. In France, however, most maternal deaths had been seen in intensive care[12]. Obviously, admission criteria to intensive care units vary, as does what constitutes intensive care. Data based on this have to be interpreted with caution, and this is not suitable as the only criterion on which to identify *near misses*.

Other interventions like the performance of intrapartum hysterectomy[16], blood transfusion or caesarean section[8] have been used to identify *near misses*. The advantage of these criteria again is the ease of identification of cases. Most would be recorded in a register in the hospital, allowing for a retrospective analysis of the cases. This is particularly useful in developing countries. However, it is prone to the same disadvantages of using intensive care as a criterion and is biased by resources available. A condition that is life threatening in a country where no appropriate response can be given may not be classified as a *near miss* and interventions such as caesarean section may often be carried out on women who are not suffering from severe acute maternal morbidity—though this may be less common in the developing than in the developed world.

Organ system dysfunction-based criteria

This system is based on the concept that there is a sequence of events leading from good health to death. The sequence is clinical insult, followed by a systemic inflammatory response syndrome, organ dysfunction, organ failure and finally death. *Near misses* would be those women with organ dysfunction and organ failure who survive. The criteria for defining a *near miss* are generic and are defined per organ system. Markers for organ system dysfunction or failure are specified, but have avoided highly technical laboratory or haemodynamic investigations. For example, renal dysfunction is defined as oliguria (<400 ml/24 h) that does not respond to fluids or diuretics, or a serum urea ≥15 mmol/l, or a creatinine ≥400 mmol/l, or the need for dialysis. Respiratory dysfunction or failure is defined as intubation and ventilation for ≥60 min for a patient not related to anaesthesia, or where the oxygen saturation is <90% for ≥60 min. The presence of any one of the markers in a pregnancy from conception to 42 days post delivery constitutes a *near miss*. Having identified the case, the primary obstetric cause can then be identified and classified. This method is the same as that of a maternal death where the death is identified then the cause allocated, but is opposite to the clinical criterion-based systems where the disease is the starting point. This system allows for identification of all critically ill women and allows for the identification of new and emerging disease priorities. It mimics the confidential enquiries into maternal death systems that a number of countries have instituted. Potentially the same system could be used to complement maternal death enquiries, as is currently occurring in Scotland[17]. The system has the advantage of being a method that a large number of developed countries can use, if agreement can be reached on the markers for organ system dysfunction and failure.

The original system included management-based markers as criteria, namely emergency hysterectomy or intensive care admission for any reason or anaesthetic accidents. This was to collect the potential *near miss* cases. For example, performing a timely hysterectomy for severe postpartum haemorrhage before losing 2.5 litres of blood or other organ failure occurred. These cases clearly represent severe morbidity but are they *near misses*? The value of including these cases has not been determined, and they might bias the sample. The indications for emergency hysterectomy might vary from site to site depending on how pro-active the consultants are. Perhaps these cases should be classified as near *near misses* and the management-based criteria left out of a *near miss* definition. It could be argued that blood loss at delivery, or clinical hypovolaemia, would be more compatible with the organ system dysfunction system than criteria based on intervention, such as transfusion, or surgery.

The organ system dysfunction has several advantages, namely:

1   Establishing the patterns of diseases causing morbidity and their relative importance.

2   Comparisons can be made providing definitions can be standardized and used in many different settings.

3   The health system is not part of the definition, so problems within the health system can be studied.

4   Cases can be flagged when they occur as a function of an ongoing audit, making it a virtually prospective audit, avoiding the problem of poor recording as illustrated earlier[11].

There are also a few disadvantages. It is dependent on a minimum level of care in the country. There must be functioning laboratories for some specific blood tests and basic critical care monitoring must be available. Retrospective identification of cases is very difficult because of the inability to identify cases from registers.

All methods of identifying *near misses* suffer from the same problem of being dependent on diligent and enthusiastic people to collect cases. Good units might detect more cases than poor units, giving a false impression of the quality of care in various areas. In some developed countries, such as Scotland, staff (usually midwives and/or obstetricians) are already given responsibility for identifying certain cases as part of risk management. The threshold for cases is usually much lower, including third degree tears, *etc.*, but should always include *near misses*. Exploration is required of whether hospital to hospital variation in *near miss* rates is simply due to small number fluctuations or whether there is differential ascertainment.

Near miss analysis as a method of assessing quality of care

The basic assumption of most outcome-audits is that by examining a few specified cases, solutions to the inadequacies found will improve not only the quality of care of similar cases but also the care of other patients in the service. The assumption is that substandard care in the patient reflects the general care of patients and is not specific to that patient. The only evidence to support this assumption is from Pandy *et al*[18]. Their group collected all maternal deaths and *near misses* due to hypertension in pregnancy from a clearly defined area in KwaZulu-Natal (South Africa). They also collected a control group of two pregnant women with hypertension per *near miss* or maternal death from the same area, delivered on the same day and matched for age and parity. The case notes were blinded and the quality of care assessed by an independent person. Substandard care was similar for the *near miss* cases and maternal deaths and uncomplicated pregnant women with hypertension.

The usefulness of analysing a few important, easily identifiable, clearly defined cases as a method of assessing the quality of care is clearly established in the case of maternal deaths. If *near misses* are added the first immediate advantage is the potential for more rapid reporting and more robust conclusions if done per disease entity. Any system of identifying *near misses* will automatically expand the database of cases for assessing maternal care.

An example of this is in Pretoria where an organ system dysfunction and failure criteria are used to identify *near misses*. During 2000–2001, a pattern shift occurred in the primary obstetric causes of *near misses*. Complications of abortions and obstetric haemorrhage became the largest cause of *near misses*, yet only two deaths per year resulting from abortion and one in 2000 and three in 2001 from obstetric haemorrhage were recorded. The number of *near misses* more than doubled from 12 to 27 cases for abortion and from 25 to 58 cases for obstetric haemorrhage. If maternal deaths alone were used to detect problems in maternal care in Pretoria, these problems would have been overlooked and remedial action considerably delayed[19].

The second advantage is the ability to compare maternal deaths with *near misses*, bringing into focus areas in the health system where there are challenges and establishing priority for action. De Bernis *et al*[20] reported on the comparison of maternal morbidity and mortality in two different populations in Senegal. In one site (Kaolack area), the women gave birth mainly in district health care centres usually assisted by traditional birth attendants, whereas in the other site (Saint-Louis), women gave birth mainly in the regional hospital and were usually assisted by midwives. The morbidity rate was lowest in the Kaolack area, but they had a significantly higher maternal mortality. Univariate and multivariate analyses showed morbidity was mainly associated with the level of training of the birth attendant in the facility deliveries. It appears that midwives in the health facilities detect more obstetric complications than traditional birth attendants. Immediate detection leads to immediate care and low fatality rates.

Another example is from Mantel et al[21] who showed that delays in transport and lack of intensive care facilities occurred significantly more in maternal deaths than women who had *near misses* in the Pretoria area. The delays were due in part to the lack of a decentralized obstetric service with the majority of maternal deaths coming from provinces outside of Pretoria. The upgrading of a hospital in one of the provinces led to a significant reduction in deaths[22].

A further advantage is the ability to examine the quality of care of a specific disease entity and identify specific problem areas such as obstetric haemorrhage as has been described above[12]. Risk factors for maternal morbidity can also be identified as shown by Waterstone et al[2] and these were remarkably similar to those of maternal death in the UK[23]. Bewley et al[24] divided the risk factors into three categories:

1   Those not amenable to change (*e.g.* race, spontaneous twinning).

2   Those that might be amenable to social change (*e.g.* maternal age, social equity).

3   Those that are within the control of health care professions (*e.g.* the care of complicated women and intervention rates).

While acknowledging the interaction between medical, political and social conditions, they suggested that the risk factors most amenable to change are obstetric interventions. They illustrate the case by giving the example of emergency caesarean section. The adjusted odds ratio of developing severe sepsis after an emergency caesarean section is particularly high. Efforts to reduce the rapidly rising caesarean section rate might be justified by the consequent reduction in severe maternal morbidity[24]. Although it could alternatively be argued that earlier caesarean section might have avoided or reduced sepsis, the benefits or otherwise of interventions can be securely established only by randomized controlled trials.

When considering whether substandard care has occurred, informal discussion may be of some value, but prior establishment of evidence-based criteria, for what would be adequate care would be preferable[26], and can be achieved for most common types of morbidity. That this approach is feasible even in small district hospitals in developing countries is encouraging[27] but it can only succeed in improving care (a) if the records are adequate, (b) if the staff feel 'ownership' of the audit ('holding up a mirror') and (c) if supplies and facilities exist to improve care. It remains to be seen whether maternal mortality will benefit. It should be noted also that as this study was focused on improving the care of women with severe acute morbidity who had actually reached hospital, it is not informative about events in the community.

In determining substandard care, those factors related to the patients' behaviour and their environment are the least accessible to analysis in women who die. Yet this is a major area where gaps in the system can be targeted and corrected. Interviews with the relatives of the dead women are fraught with difficulties and the data obtained not reliable. Inclusion of *near misses* provides an opportunity of obtaining this information on behaviour and environmental factors. For example, in interviews of all the *near misses* that occurred in the Pretoria region[21], some clear barriers to access of services were identified. Seventy-nine percent of women did not have a telephone at home or a private car. The majority of women (58%) did not know that the clinic closest to them was closed after hours. On average, the nearest local 24-h services was 45 min away and 82% had to use a taxi to get to that service. Patients bypassed local services and went directly to the tertiary hospitals because they apparently did not know of their existence or did not trust their quality of care, thereby delaying treatment that could have prevented the *near miss*.

A number of authors have suggested establishing an index of sorts so that the changes can be identified. Bewley *et al*[24] suggested the Morbidity to Mortality Ratio. Bouvier-Colle *et al*[12] described the Lethality Rate, which is the ratio of maternal deaths to all obstetric patients admitted for treatment or surveillance to an intensive care unit or the closest equivalent surgical or medical resuscitation or critical care unit in the region. Vandecruys *et al*[22] described the Mortality Index, which was defined as the number of maternal deaths divided by the sum of maternal deaths and *near misses*. All these indices have the advantage of comparing units and of plotting changes in a particular unit over time. For this to be achieved, consensus on the criteria used to identify *near misses* must be agreed and there must be constancy in their use. The advantages for this can be illustrated by the following example. Sites in Bloemfontein, Pretoria and Soweto in South Africa achieved agreement on the criteria. This allowed comparison of Mortality Indices for various conditions at the three sites. Surprisingly large differences occurred in the three sites with generally two sites (not consistently the same sites) being similar and one site significantly higher. Investigation into the differences showed variations in management protocols and the way the health system functioned[25]. The Pretoria region has used the same definitions of *near miss* for the past 5 years. Changes in rates of *near misses* and maternal deaths and

Table 1 Comparison of the pattern changes in rates of *near misses* plus maternal deaths in Pretoria over 5 years

Primary obstetric causes	1997–9	2000	2001	2002
Direct				
Abortion	152	87	169	228
Ectopic pregnancy	50	51	25	133
Antepartum haemorrhage	73	43	125	76
Postpartum haemorrhage	96	137	238	228
Hypertension	84	108	138	133
Pregnancy-related sepsis	15	43	75	57
Embolism	8	7	13	6
Anaesthetic complications	27	36	13	13
Indirect				
Non-pregnancy-related infections	23	58	25	63
Pre-existing maternal disease	46	72	50	51

Rates expressed per 100,000 births.

Table 2 Comparison of the changes in Mortality Indices in Pretoria over 5 years

Primary obstetric causes	1997–9	2000	2001	2002
Direct				
Abortion	15	18	8	2.7
Ectopic pregnancy	0	16	0	4.5
Antepartum haemorrhage	0	0	5	0
Postpartum haemorrhage	4	5	5	5.2
Hypertension	9.1	20	23	8.7
Pregnancy-related sepsis	50	0	0	0
Embolism	100	100	50	100
Anaesthetic complications	0	0	0	0
Indirect				
Non-pregnancy-related infections	50	76	24	37.5
Pre-existing maternal disease	25	26	24	11
Total	14	19	11	10

the Mortality Indices are shown in Tables 1 and 2. In Pretoria, preventing complications for abortions, obstetric haemorrhage and hypertension are the priority concerns despite the fact that the highest Mortality Indices are for embolism, which is rare but commonly fatal.

Conclusion

Confidential enquiries into maternal deaths have been associated with decreases in maternal deaths, but in developed countries, maternal deaths are now rare and the relevance of the information gleaned from the occasional maternal death to the general population is becoming distant. The incorporation of *near misses* into the confidential enquiry systems might allow for more relevant data on maternal care being made applicable. Hall[17] listed several reasons for their inclusion.

1 Larger numbers lead to more robust conclusions.

2 More rapid reporting on maternal care issues (because of the larger number of cases).

3 Useful lessons learnt from *near misses* will reinforce the lessons learnt when these cases previously died.

4 *Near misses* will provide relevant controls for maternal deaths, since presumably most women who die pass through a phase of organ dysfunction before dying.

5 Provided an ethical solution can be found to the confidentiality problem, the *near misses* can be interviewed providing valuable information on the risk factors and substandard care.

6 Obstetric requirements for intensive care can be quantified.

7 Comparative ratios/indices can be calculated.

However, before such a system is introduced, consensus will need to be attained on the criteria used to identify a *near miss*.

References

1 Macfarlane A. Enquiries into maternal deaths during the 20th century. In: *Why Mothers Die 1997–1999: The Confidential Enquiries into Maternal Deaths in the United Kingdom*. Department of Health, Welsh Office, Scottish Home and Health Department, Department of Heath and Social Sciences, Northern Ireland. London: RCOG Press, 2001; 346–57

2 Waterstone M, Bewley S, Wolfe C. Incidence and predictors of severe obstetric morbidity: case-control study. *BMJ* 2001; **322**: 1089–94

3 Introduction and key findings. In: *Why Mothers Die 1997–1999: The Confidential Enquiries into Maternal Deaths in the United Kingdom*. Department of Health, Welsh Office, Scottish Home and Health Department, Department of Heath and Social Sciences, Northern Ireland. London: RCOG Press, 2001; 22–45

4 De Swiet M. Cardiac disease. In: *Why Mothers Die 1997–1999: The Confidential Enquiries into Maternal Deaths in the United Kingdom*. Department of Health, Welsh Office, Scottish Home and Health Department, Department of Heath and Social Sciences, Northern Ireland. London: RCOG Press, 2001; 153–64

5 *Measuring Reproductive Morbidity*. Report of a technical working group. Geneva: World Health Organization (unpublished document WHO/MCH/90.4; available on request from Family and Community Health, World Health Organization, 1211 Geneva 27, Switzerland)

6 Nashef SAM. What is a near miss? *Lancet* 2003; **361**: 180–1

7 Filippi V, Ronsmans C, Gandaho T, Graham W, Alihonou E, Santos P. Women's reports of severe (near miss) obstetric complications in Benin. *Stud Fam Plann* 2000; **31**: 309–24

8 Prual A, Bouvier-Colle M-H, de Bernis L, Breat G. Severe maternal morbidity from direct obstetric causes in West Africa: incidence and case fatality rates. *Bull WHO* 2000; **78**: 593–602

9 Mantel GD, Buchmann E, Rees H, Pattinson RC. Severe acute maternal morbidity: a pilot study of a definition for a near-miss. *Br J Obstet Gynaecol* 1998; **105**: 985–90

10 Ronsmans C, Filippi V. Reviewing severe maternal morbidity: learning from women who survive life-threatening complications. In: *Beyond the Numbers*. Geneva: World Health Organization; In press

11 Bouvier-Colle M-H, Joud DOE, Varnoux N *et al*. Evaluation of the quality of care for severe obstetrical haemorrhage in three French regions. *Br J Obstet Gynaecol* 2001; **108**: 898–903

12 Bouvier-Colle M-H, Salanave B, Ancel PY *et al*. Obstetric patients in intensive care units and maternal mortality. Regional Teams for the Survey. *Eur J Obstet Gynecol Reprod Biol* 1996; **65**: 121–5

13 Baskett TF, Sternadel J. Maternal intensive care and near-miss mortality in obstetrics. *Br J Obstet Gynaecol* 1998; **105**: 981–4

14 Fitzpatrick C, Halligan A, McKenna P, Coughlan BM, Darling MR, Phelan D. Near miss maternal mortality (NMM). *Ir Med J* 1992; **85**: 37

15 Willatts SM. Intensive care. In: *Why Mothers Die 1997–1999: The Confidential Enquiries into Maternal Deaths in the United Kingdom*. Department of Health, Welsh Office, Scottish Home and Health Department, Department of Heath and Social Sciences, Northern Ireland. London: RCOG Press, 2001; 309–16

16 Nasrat HA, Youssef MH, Marzoogi A, Talab F. Near miss obstetric morbidity in an inner city hospital in Saudi Arabia. *East Mediterranean Health J* 1999; **5**: 717–26

17 Hall MH. Near misses and severe maternal morbidity. In: *Why Mothers Die 1997–1999: The Confidential Enquiries into Maternal Deaths in the United Kingdom*. Department of Health, Welsh Office, Scottish Home and Health Department, Department of Heath and Social Sciences, Northern Ireland. London: RCOG Press, 2001; 323–5

18 Pandy M, Mantel GD, Moodley J. Audit of severe acute morbidity in hypertensive pregnancies. Abstracts of the 28th South African Society of Obstetricians and Gynaecologists Congress, Durban, 6–10 April 2003. Durban: University of Natal Press

19 Cochet L, Pattinson RC, Macdonald AP. Severe acute maternal morbidity and maternal death audit. A rapid diagnostic tool for evaluating maternal care. *S Afr Med J*; In press

20 De Bernis L, Dumont A, Bouillin D, Gueye A, Dompnier J-P, Bouvier-Colle M-H. Maternal morbidity and mortality in two different populations in Senegal: a prospective study (MOMA survey). *Br J Obstet Gynaecol* 2000; **107**: 68–74

21 Mantel GD, Pattinson RC, Macdonald AP. *Maternal Mortality and Severe Acute Morbidity (Near Misses) in the Pretoria Region: 1/2/1997–31/1/1999*. Report to Gauteng Department of Health, 1999

22 Vandecruys H, Pattinson RC, Macdonald AP, Mantel G. Severe acute maternal morbidity and mortality in the Pretoria Academic Complex: Changing patterns over 4 years. *Eur J Obstet Gynaecol Reprod Biol* 2001; **102**: 6–10

23 Lewis G. Risk factors for maternal death in the UK. In: MacLean AB, Neilson JP (eds) *Maternal Morbidity and Mortality*. London: RCOG Press, 2002; 119–31

24 Bewley S, Wolfe C, Waterstone M. Severe morbidity in the UK. In: MacLean AB, Neilson JP (eds) *Maternal Morbidity and Mortality*. London: RCOG Press, 2002; 132–46

25 Pattinson RC. Major maternal morbidity in South Africa. In: MacLean AB, Neilson JP (eds) *Maternal Morbidity and Mortality*. London: RCOG Press, 2002; 147–57

26 Graham W, Wagaarachchi P, Penney G, McCaw-Binns A, Antwi KY, Hall MH. Criteria for clinical audit of the quality of hospital-based obstetric care in developing countries. *WHO Bull* 2000; **78**: 614–820

27 Wagaarachchi P, Graham WJ, Penney G, McCaw-Binns A, Antwi KY, Hall MH. Holding up a mirror: changing obstetric practice through criterion-based clinical audit in developing countries. *Int J Gynaecol Obstet* 2001; **74**: 119–30

Useful websites

www.aed.org
Academy for Educational Development.

www.b-lineproductions.co.uk
The website of B-Line Productions, a specialist producer of videos on birth, breast-feeding, weaning, etc.

www.comminit.com
Communication Initiative Network.

www.engenderhealth.org

www.fhi.org
New website from Family Health International, includes HIV/AIDS, reproductive health and family planning information, with a focus on the welfare of young people and overviews of country programmes.

www.infoforhealth.org
New resource on family planning and reproductive health from the INFO Project of Johns Hopkins Bloomberg School of Public Health. Includes latest research findings on topics relevant to WHO's family planning guidance.

www.internationalmidwives.org
The website for the International Confederation of Midwives which aims to advance worldwide the aims and aspirations of midwives in the attainment of improved outcomes for women in their childbearing years, their newborn and their families wherever they reside.

www.ippf.org
The website of the International Planned Parenthood Federation, a UK registered charity and the largest voluntary organization in the world to be concerned with family planning and sexual and reproductive health.

www.nct-online.org
The website for the National Childbirth Trust, which offers support in pregnancy, childbirth and early parenthood.

www.reproductiverights.org
Website from The Centre for Reproductive Rights, a non-profit legal advocacy organization, includes 'Reproductive Freedom News'.

www.reproline.jhu.edu
Reproductive Health Online.

www.talcuk.org
The website for Teaching-aids At Low Cost, a charity which supplies low-cost healthcare, training and teaching materials.

www.whiteribbonalliance.org
The White Ribbon Alliance for Safe Motherhood.

www.who.int/reproductive-health/mpr
Making Pregnancy Safer website.

Index